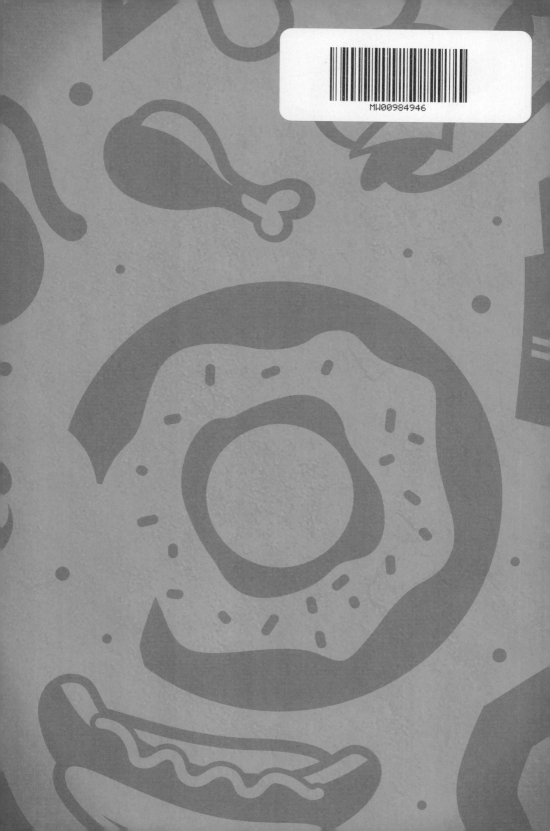

# What people are saying about *Eating Yourself Sick*

"Since our undergraduate days at Syracuse University, I knew Joe Galati was going to make a huge impact. His passion, dedication, and drive to make the world a healthier place come though in every page of this wonderful and engaging book. Physician, radio host, and now author— what a thrill to read his life's work in *Eating Yourself Sick*. It's powerful, compelling, and a great read for anyone who strives to maximize their health and wellness."

## Chuck Garcia
Amazon best selling author of *A Climb to the TOP*

"As a primary care physician, I see first-hand the devastating effects of obesity and diabetes. As a hospital executive, every day I witness the toll that obesity and diabetes has on chronic disease, with a substantial percentage of hospitalized patients suffering the impact of these diseases.

And as the leader of an organization that invests in its employees' health, I see the impact of chronic disease on them and their families. It is important to discuss obesity and the role it plays in our health, so I applaud Dr. Galati for his insightful and thought-provoking discussion of these issues."

## Marc L. Boom, MD
President, Chief Executive Officer, Houston Methodist Hospital

"With clarity and insight, Dr. Galati masterfully defines the obesity epidemic and links this condition with diabetes, liver and cardiovascular disease. His easy to understand descriptions and his practical approach makes this book a must read to raise heath IQ across the country. As a cardiologist, husband, father and son, this wonderfully written book will guide my patients and family on the rationale behind adopting a healthier life style."

## Jerry D. Estep, MD, FACC, FASE
Associate Professor of Clinical Cardiology
Houston Methodist Institute of Academic Medicine
Section Head of Heart Transplant & Mechanical Circulatory Support,
Division of Heart Failure
Medical Director, Heart Transplant & LVAD Program
Methodist DeBakey Heart & Vascular Center
Houston Methodist Hospital

"In this highly readable and approachable book, Dr. Galati brings experience derived from his career as a renowned expert in liver disease together with his skills as a communicator to bear on a disorder that is a modern epidemic. In a style that is lucid and understandable, yet never condescending to the reader, he not only takes us through the causes and impacts of the modern obesity epidemic, but he also provides solutions that are realistic and attainable."

## Eamonn M. M. Quigley, MD, FRCP, FACP, MACG, FRCPI
David M Underwood Chair of Medicine in Digestive Disorders,
Co-Director, Lynda K and David M Underwood Center for Digestive Disorders,
Chief, Gastroenterology and Hepatology,
Professor of Medicine, Institute of Academic Medicine, Houston Methodist Hospital;
Professor of Medicine, Weill Cornell Medical College;
Adjunct Professor of Medicine, Texas A and M Health Sciences Center College of Medicine

"With an easy, flowing style reminiscent of his conversations on his syndicated radio show, Dr. Galati demystifies what most people do not know or choose to ignore about our modern diets. Metabolic overload, a result of not only how much we eat, but also what we choose to eat, is a major driving force for the diseases we see today. In clinical practice, we see increased blood pressure, increased prevalence of kidney disorders, and skyrocketing rates of heart disease. Today, chronic kidney disease and fatty liver disease are reaching epidemic proportions in many communities and threatens not just the health of individuals, but also the very health of the population and economic growth of many countries. Dr. Galati, in his smooth, elegant style, describes the origins of these problems and provides— through his description—the potential solutions. As a practitioner dedicated to the eradication of advanced organ failure, Dr. Galati's book is a must read for everyone, particularly those raising young families where having this awareness may actually change the future."

### A. Osama Gaber, MD, FACS

J.C. Walter Jr. Presidential Distinguished Chair & Director, J.C. Walter Jr. Transplant Center
Professor of Surgery, Institute for Academic Medicine
Program Director, Transplant Surgery Residency, Department of Surgery
Houston Methodist Hospital
Weill Cornell Medical College

"The drivers of obesity are complex—diets high in sugars and carbohydrates, processed foods, over-eating, lack of exercise, certain medications, underlying illnesses, and alterations in the absorption of nutrients all play important roles to a person's health. As you can imagine, the vast number of causes for obesity does not allow for a one-size-fits-all solution.

Obesity keeps bad company. High blood pressure, diabetes, sleep apnea, and heart disease are just a few medical conditions associated with being overweight. The impact of obesity on our collective health is devastating, and the number of children afflicted with this condition are increasing with alarming frequency.

It is time to take control of this epidemic. All of us need to view obesity as a disease rather than a personal flaw and attack it with the same rigor as other medical conditions like cancer and HIV. Physicians and other healthcare professionals can help in the battle but they will only be successful if our patients and their families join the fight. Together, we can tackle one of the most important epidemics of this century."

### Joseph G. Rogers, MD

Professor of Medicine
Division of Cardiology
Interim Chair, Department of Medicine
Duke University School of Medicine

# EATING YOURSELF
# SICK
## JOSEPH S. GALATI, MD

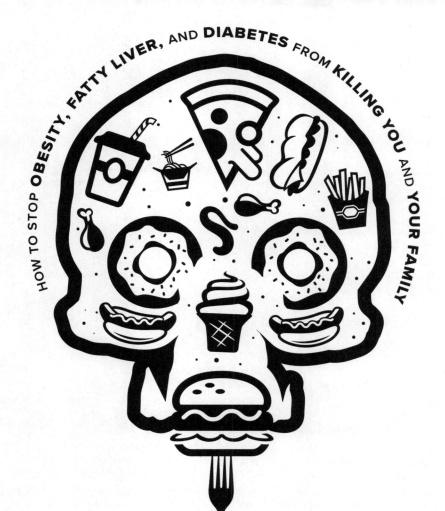

HOW TO STOP **OBESITY**, FATTY **LIVER**, AND **DIABETES** FROM **KILLING YOU** AND **YOUR FAMILY**

EATING YOURSELF

# SICK

## JOSEPH S. GALATI, MD

*Advantage*®

Published by Advantage, Charleston, South Carolina.
Member of Advantage Media Group.

ADVANTAGE is a registered trademark, and the Advantage colophon is a trademark of Advantage Media Group, Inc.

Printed in the United States of America.

10  9  8  7  6  5  4  3  2  1

ISBN: 978-1-59932-914-7
LCCN: 2018935791

Cover and layout designed by George Stevens.

This publication is designed to provide accurate and authoritative information in regard to the subject matter covered. It is sold with the understanding that the publisher is not engaged in rendering legal, accounting, or other professional services. If legal advice or other expert assistance is required, the services of a competent professional person should be sought.

 Advantage Media Group is proud to be a part of the Tree Neutral® program. Tree Neutral offsets the number of trees consumed in the production and printing of this book by taking proactive steps such as planting trees in direct proportion to the number of trees used to print books. To learn more about Tree Neutral, please visit **www.treeneutral.com**.

Advantage Media Group is a publisher of business, self-improvement, and professional development books and online learning. We help entrepreneurs, business leaders, and professionals share their Stories, Passion, and Knowledge to help others Learn & Grow. Do you have a manuscript or book idea that you would like us to consider for publishing? Please visit **advantagefamily.com** or call **1.866.775.1696**.

To Geraldine: The love of my life, best friend, and hiking partner. You've been by my side throughout this journey. Thank you for always understanding.

To Joseph and Elizabeth: No father could be prouder of his children than I am. Always remain faithful to your dreams.

To Mom and Dad: The lifetime of conversations we shared in the kitchen remains with me today, as vivid as ever. They have been a constant source of inspiration, direction, and wisdom I'll never forget.

To Celeste Zerbarini: Thank you for your love; you have shared the 3 Fs with your family so very well.

To Anne Galati Campolieta: Through your devastating illness, you taught me humility and courage as a young physician.

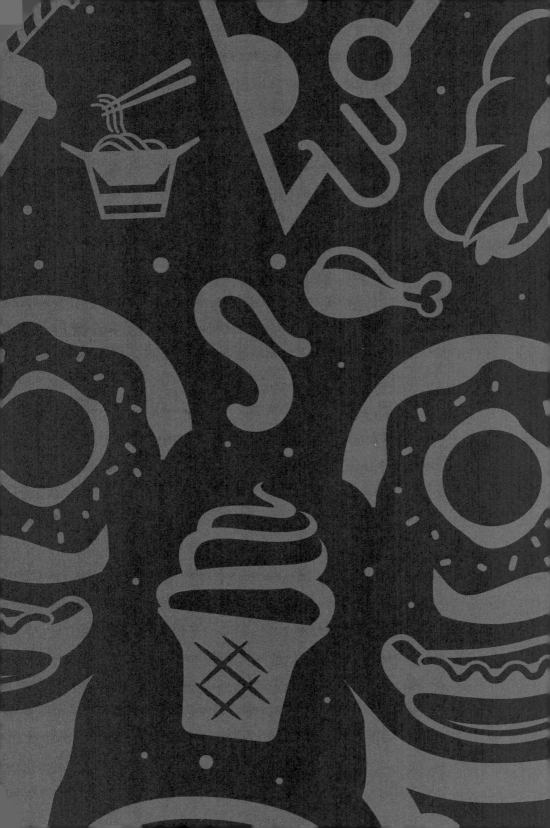

# ACKNOWLEDGMENTS

**I have always** said that when you look back at your life, it is a patchwork of people and experiences sewn together. For me, I have been blessed with a large number of friends and colleagues who have had a meaningful impact on me. This book is a culmination of all my life experiences to date, and the lessons I've learned from those closest to me.

First and foremost, I'd like to thank all the patients I have cared for over the past thirty years. It is a tremendous responsibility to receive trust from patients and their families to care for a loved one with a serious illness. I have learned invaluable lessons from all of you. Allowing me to be a part of the good and bad times has been a privilege—one I never have taken for granted.

I must also recognize the unsung heroes in transplantation, the organ donors and their families who made the conscious decision to donate the organs of a loved one to a total stranger, allowing someone else a chance to continue living. There are truly no words to express this gratitude for the gift of life to others.

Thank you to all of my friends on Long Island and at Holy Trinity High School. You all played an important role in who I am today, and the experiences we shared for many years were indeed formative in what I do today.

To all of my friends and colleagues at the University of Nebraska Medical Center and in Houston at the Texas Medical Center, including Drs. Michael Sorrell, Rowen Zetterman, Eamonn Quigley, Bud Shaw, Alan Langnas, Howard Monsour, R. Patrick Wood, Claire Ozaki, Mark Ghobrial, Osama Gaber, Victor Ankoma-Sey, and Isaac Raijman. The care and compassion you have all shown toward your patients has been exemplary. You are all great role models to me.

Thank you to all the nurses and liver transplant coordinators I have worked with over the years. Your dedication to some of the sickest patients anywhere on earth has been amazing to observe.

Thank you to all the staff, past and current, at the Liver Specialists of Texas and the Metabolic and Fatty Liver Center. You have impacted thousands of lives for the better.

To my Entrepreneurs Organization forum mates, George, Frank, Tom, Royce, Jeb, Adam, Bill, David, and Jarred—your support, encouragement, and honesty has been invaluable.

To Al Danto, for all of the streetlight conversations we had and giving me the courage to change course.

To Deborah Keener Brown, for meeting me on a rainy Sunday afternoon and passing on my radio demo to Eddie Martini at Clear Channel/iHeart Radio. You have both allowed me to share my passion on the radio through all these years.

To Dave Dillon, who gave me the moniker "physician communicator."

To Ray Schilens at the Radio Lounge, for all the technical support to get *Your Health First* on the air every week.

To Fred Haubenreich, who loaned me his Nikon F camera and patiently taught me the art of photography and black-and-white film chemistry when I was fourteen years old.

To Chuck Garcia, "To us and all that we represent."

To Regina Roths, who assisted me in the manuscript preparation, who shared her own personal family experience with liver disease.

And to those who reviewed the early stages of the manuscript and provided me with valuable clarity, especially Madeline Drake, Kathy Fenelon, Dr. Archana Sadhu, and Dr. Eamonn Quigley.

# TABLE OF CONTENTS

# INTRODUCTION
# Family, Faith, And Food

**My mother was** an amazing woman who lived a full life. She passed away in late January 2016, just weeks shy of her eighty-eighth birthday.

During the prayer service at O'Shea's Funeral Home on Long Island, I mentally cobbled together a few thoughts about Mom to share with our friends, neighbors, and relatives she had touched in some way.

As Deacon Bob O'Donovan of our church called on me, I stepped forward, sticky note in hand with only three words written on it: family, faith, and food. Those three words really encapsulated the essence of what my mother represented—love of family, an intense faith she shared with us all, and the love of preparing food for family and visitors at her kitchen table. I spoke through the impulse to cry—smiles and nods from family and friends gave me the encouragement to carry on and complete my five-minute tribute. And as I spoke, I realized the things that my mother valued—family, faith, and food—were also central to my own life.

I had an amazing childhood, growing up on the south shore of Long Island in the 1960s and '70s. My Brooklyn-native father was an army medic in World War II who participated in campaigns in North Africa and Italy and had received a Bronze Star and Purple Heart. He also had a long career in pharmaceutical sales. The ultimate "people person" and communicator, his personality and speaking skills greatly influenced me. My mother, meanwhile, grew up in Astoria, Queens and, like my father, was also the product of Italian and Sicilian immigrants. She graduated from high school and became an executive secretary in the pharmaceutical and medical fields.

With both of my parents in the health field, I was exposed early to the world of medicine, and could often be found thumbing through the *Journal of the American Medical Association* (JAMA), cutting out pictures of tumors and X-rays from the journal pages, and taping them to my bedroom wall. My father had a vast library of 8mm Technicolor movies that were used as part of the available sales-training tools for physicians and vividly showed various surgeries showcasing the various products being sold. Watching those silent movies at around five years old made me realize I wanted to get involved in medicine.

My sisters, Anne and Celeste, and I (the "three Gs," as we were known), had a great upbringing. My parents were early adopters of the now popular "work-life balance" idea, passing on career opportunities to keep our family whole. Dad had multiple opportunities for promotions with the pharmaceutical giant he worked for, Warner Lambert. But each opportunity would mean relocating the family, so my parents opted to decline each one, considering the impact such moves would have on the family. Although they would have made more money, the opportunities would have required my dad to travel and be away from the family for extended periods. To this day, at ninety-three years old, Dad has no regrets about his career choices. He and my mom agreed: The most important thing was a strong family, and that meant togetherness. Maintaining the familiarity of our community, school, and church was viewed as the key to our happiness.

Communication was also key for creating strong family bonds, and the primary venue for that was the kitchen table. Whenever we were together, whether at the kitchen table or elsewhere, there was conversation and storytelling. My parents often shared what they experienced at work or in conversations they had with others around town, and their stories contained both facts and parables—they always conveyed a takeaway message. This was not a chance event but rather part of their grand plan in raising three children. The stories were usually rooted in faith, and acted as a moral compass on how we should react to a situation, or how we should treat someone. Raised Roman Catholic, my sisters and I attended our parish grade school and later the Diocesan Catholic high school. We attended church every week, and the majority of our extracurricular time was spent in numerous parish activities, with mom acting as the full-time "taxi driver" for us and our friends.

My mother didn't smoke or drink; her drug of choice was cooking. She considered cooking for the family to be one of the most important responsibilities of a mother. She was the first one out of bed each school morning and would head to the kitchen to prepare a hot breakfast for us. We always had lunches from home (we never bought the school cafeteria meal), and dinner each night was a planned menu. She was a self-taught, Renaissance woman when it came to wellness and nutrition, and she understood the value of eating a balanced and fresh diet. "You are what you eat," was a phrase she commonly used, and she often chastised others who let their families eat the early versions of processed, manufactured food that was stripped of nutrients. "Eat that garbage and you'll be the size of a whale in a year," she'd quip. She truly believed the responsibility of the parent was to ensure the family ate well; *she believed creating a healthful environment was first and foremost the responsibility of a parent.*

As a result, no one in my family ever had health or weight issues; diabetes didn't stand a chance on my mom's watch. Back then, in the early 1970s, mom was the head coach in her crusade for good health. She considered cooking a team sport. We each had an assigned duty, and with proper training and success, we moved up the ranks. Each of us started off chopping garlic and onions, then moved on to pressing tomatoes, then slicing eggplants and zucchini. Mom hovered over us like an assembly-line foreman, ensuring pieces were just the right size, not too big or small. Luckily, in mom's kitchen there were do-overs—lots of them! If a cut wasn't up to standard, she'd have us do it again while she supervised. Her instruction wasn't punitive; she was simply training us to appreciate the value and beauty of a home-cooked meal done right. Nutrition and wellness was stressed at every opportunity, and she was dead serious about it.

The concept of family, faith, and food—the "3 Fs"—has had a tremendous impact on who I am today. The lessons I learned in that small Long Island home are lessons I strive to replicate with my own family. My wife and I support our children emotionally and spiritually, and ensure their health and wellness is maintained with a solid, nutritional underpinning. Like my mother, I enjoy preparing fresh meals at home and getting everyone involved in the food preparation process.

Teaching children how to cook and feel comfortable in the kitchen is an important facet of wellness, and a responsibility parents should take seriously. The dereliction of this responsibility, like outsourcing it to a drive-through window, is a major contributing factor to obesity and all the disastrous complications of metabolic syndrome. Despite the medical breakthroughs in the past fifty years, we are now faced with the reality that the children of today will not live as long as their parents. Obesity, diabetes, fatty liver, and cardiovascular disease will destroy the productivity and livelihoods of an entire generation. Who in their right mind finds this acceptable? Where is the outrage?

As a physician, the "3 Fs" are on my mind daily, and I question my patients regularly on how they view them, albeit in a somewhat roundabout fashion. I inquire about their families—who's at home and the makeup of children and extended family members who live under the same roof. Why am I so interested? Because I have found that the lack of family cohesiveness is a risk factor for damaging health habits which increase the risk of disease. Research has clearly indicated the gradual erosion of the family unit in the United States has resulted in numerous social and health consequences. As the family unit fragments—the result of divorce, single parents, and working parents—everyone is too busy to stop and place any emphasis on the job of meal planning and cooking. While attention to millennials, who prefer take-out, has been stressed in the news, adults of all ages are too rushed to cook, and simply are not interested in cooking. Eating has become a "fetch-for-yourself" activity, and it is viewed as more of a nuisance than an important part of the day and source of good nutrition. These factors and more have resulted in a society of poor food choices that have ultimately led to an obesity epidemic.

As for faith, I'm referring to it in the most general sense, as in a respect for self and others who surround us. A faithful individual spreads optimism, not gloom. It is taking responsibility for our children, spouses, and friends, a large part of which is thinking about what we feed them. That faithful responsibility my mother commanded in our kitchen has merit in today's society.

And when it comes to food, I ask my patients who in the household prepares the weekly menu (if one exists), who shops, who cooks, and what skills they have in the kitchen. I'm not asking questions to embarrass anyone but rather to evaluate what challenges they face in preparing healthful food.

Those challenges include trying to understand what "nutrition" means in today's food choices. Over the past thirty years, the food industry has made tremendous strides in food safety, selection, shelf life, and availability. However, the majority of these new food items are manufactured products with many nutritional benefits stripped out, like fiber, instead adding things we don't need. They are high in fat, salt, and sugar, all factors contributing to global obesity—and to disease. While most health professionals suggest their patients "eat more fruits and vegetables," the sad reality is that many patients are incapable of even identifying fruits and vegetables, let alone properly cook them. As a result, they head to the inner aisles of their favorite mega-supermarket and pick up something already prepared, something loaded with everything their physician would actually prefer they avoid.

As a hepatologist, a physician who specializes in the liver, including all facets of diseases affecting the liver such as fatty liver and metabolic syndrome, every day I see the ill effects poor eating has on the human body. Every day, I take the time to have technical and emotionally complicated, in-depth discussions with people who have or are on the path to life-threatening illness—and most of the time it's because of how they've viewed nutrition and eating. What I do is rewarding, recharging work. In my daily practice, I am one voice seeing patients every day, however, through my radio show "Your Health First," which I've broadcasted since 2003, I put together this book to help people understand this message: Your lifestyle is killing you and your children, but by taking responsibility for the "3 Fs," you can turn things around. If we take seriously the health issues that confront us as a nation—realizing that the obesity epidemic and all of its devastating effects will leave none of our families untouched—we can reduce the suffering ahead.

This book is the culmination of thirty years in medicine, tens of thousands of interviews with patients and their families, and lifelong learning in the kitchen and at the dining table. I'm going to share with you what my mother instilled in me, and the lessons I have learned since, about healthy eating and the benefits of cooking for yourself and your family.

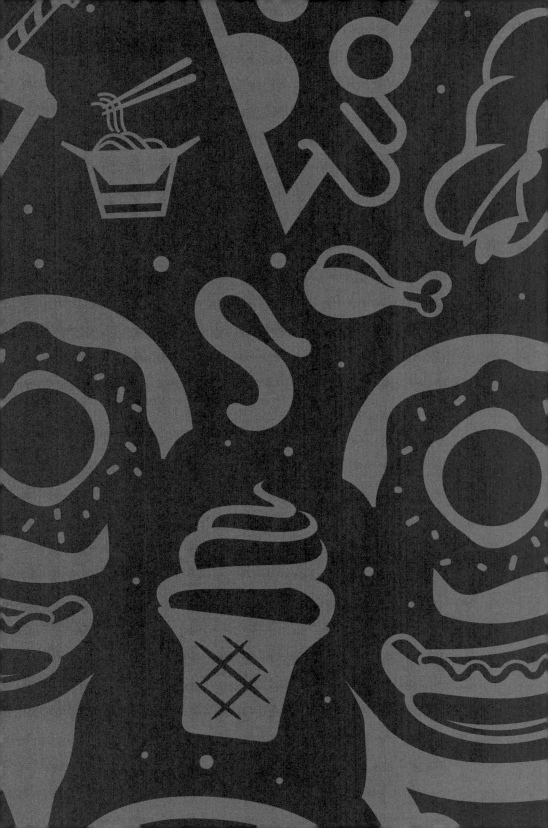

# CHAPTER 1

# Understanding Obesity-Related Disease: Your Wake-Up Call

→ *A Low Health IQ*
→ *The Other MS*
→ *The Lead Player: Obesity*
→ *There's No Such Thing as "a Touch of Diabetes"*
→ *Cardiovascular Disease*
→ *Your Fatty Liver*
→ *Gastroesophageal Reflux Disease (GERD)*
→ *Obstructive Sleep Apnea*
→ *Reproductive Health and the ED Connection*
→ *The Cancer Link*
→ *And Then There's Depression*
→ *The Cost of Obesity—Everyone is Effected*
→ *It's About Priorities*

**When Laura was** in her mid-twenties, she went to her primary care physician, complaining of bloating and abdominal distress, mild bouts of nausea and gas, and occasional constipation. Her primary care doctor ordered lab tests and an ultrasound to see if there was a problem with her gallbladder or pancreas. When her tests showed elevated liver enzymes and an enlarged liver, he referred her to me.

During my consultation with her, she nonchalantly told me that she had been diagnosed with fatty liver ten years earlier.

"What were you told to do at that time?" I asked.

"Just lose some weight," she replied, shrugging her shoulders.

At the time, Laura was significantly obese. She was taking medication for high blood pressure and had unfounded concerns that the medication would harm her liver. She also had high blood glucose levels, indicating she was on the doorstep of diabetes, but she wasn't doing anything to keep her blood sugar in check.

Her family history of ill health compounded her situation: her mother was diabetic and had died of cirrhosis, her father was an alcoholic, and her siblings were overweight. Laura herself had gestational diabetes for two of her three pregnancies, placing her at high risk for the eventual development of type 2 diabetes.

Her lifestyle wasn't optimum for good health. She worked at a Texas Gulf Coast chemical plant, never exercised, and ate out for most of her meals because she was too tired to cook or clean up afterward. Her partner and children had similar eating habits. Most of the time, the whole family ate mostly processed and fast food: cold cereals, frozen pizza, burgers and fries, ice cream, and cake. On the rare nights that Laura did cook dinner, the meal typically consisted of fried meat, canned or frozen vegetables, and a boxed side dish. Those nights, at least the family ate together—but while sitting in the living room watching TV.

Laura's story is all too common, and it doesn't discriminate by age, race, religion, profession, or other factors. I see Laura every day in people from all walks of life, from executives in their fifties to working parents in their thirties and forties to retirees age sixty and over. On any given day, I have the same conversation with at least ten people as I had with Laura: I tell them that without proper nutritional food choices, regular exercise, and a healthier lifestyle, they're putting themselves at risk for serious disease, and even premature death.

## A Low Health IQ

In talking to Laura about nutrition, I found that her biggest problem was the same one suffered by Americans nationwide: she had what I call a low health IQ. She simply didn't understand how her body worked and what it needed to stay healthy. She didn't understand the harm that obesity, diabetes, high cholesterol, fatty liver disease, and high blood pressure wreak on the body's systems. She didn't understand that she was making poor food and lifestyle choices. And thanks to food-label confusion, store aisles stocked with unhealthy choices, and streets lined with fast-food restaurants, she didn't even know what healthy food was.

> **Your Health IQ**
> Do you realize that gestational diabetes in a twenty-five-year old woman puts you at risk for type 2 diabetes at fifty years old?

On my weekly radio show, *Your Health First*, my mission is to *raise the health IQ of my audience one listener at a time*, and with this book, I'm hoping to reach even more people. I hope to help you better understand your body and the role nutrition plays in good health. I hope to help you see that, as I mentioned in the introduction, the three Fs—family, faith, and food—are key to you and your family living your best life.

## The Other MS

Laura's story illustrates what happens when multiple issues affect a person's health and create a condition that is quickly taking center stage as a world health crisis: metabolic syndrome.

Metabolic syndrome was first described in 1988 by Gerald Reaven, an American endocrinologist, who found that there were various contributing factors in people at high risk for cardiovascular disease, heart attack, and stroke. What I have termed *the other MS*, metabolic syndrome is a combination of disorders: truncal obesity, diabetes (or insulin resistance), cardiovascular disease, elevated cholesterol, and nonalcoholic fatty liver (NAFL). On its own, each disorder in this cast of characters can wreak havoc on the body. Together, they can even spell death.

| Metabolic Syndrome ||
| --- | --- |
| Truncal obesity (aka belly fat) | Elevated cholesterol or triglycerides |
| High blood pressure | Fatty liver |
| Pre-diabetes and type-2 diabetes ||

*Metabolic syndrome is a collection of conditions that occur together, increasing your risk of heart disease, stroke, diabetes, and cirrhosis. Having more than one of these could increase your risk even greater.*

Since up to 25 percent of the world's adults have metabolic syndrome, it's imperative to identify these people now so that early lifestyle interventions and treatment can begin. That is the way to prevent metabolic syndrome from becoming an established epidemic, as type 2 diabetes and cardiovascular disease already are.[1]

## The Lead Player: Obesity

In the cast of characters that make up *the other MS*, one takes center stage: obesity. In fact, it could be argued that, without obesity, the other disorders would not exist.

According to the World Health Organization, obesity has more than doubled worldwide since 1980. In 2014, more than 1.9 billion adults were overweight, including 600 million considered to be obese. Those overweight comprised 39 percent of the adult population, one-third of all people age eighteen and over.[2]

Some forty-two million children age four and under were also overweight or obese.[3] Since 1980, the rates of obesity have tripled in youth, ages two to nineteen, while the numbers of obese six- to eleven-year-olds has doubled, and obese teenagers quadrupled from 5 to 20 percent.[4] There are significant racial and ethnic inequalities in those numbers. Latinos and blacks, for example, become obese earlier, faster, and more frequently than whites and Asian.[5] Once thought of as a problem only affecting high-income countries, today obesity is on the rise in low- and middle-income areas of the world. In fact, the World Health Organization (WHO) reports that, worldwide, overweight and obesity now accounts for more deaths than underweight.[6]

In a recent *New England Journal of Medicine* article, childhood obesity has been shown to be a strong indicator of obesity at age thirty-five. Obese two-year-olds have a better than 50 percent chance of being obese at thirty-five, showing the powerful predictive value of obesity at a young age. The discussion about obesity, as a result, needs to start even sooner, and is not just a problem of the over-fifty club.[7]

So, obesity is a trend going in the wrong direction. What happened? Well, a number of factors.

## Eating More Grains

In 1985, the National Heart, Lung and Blood Institute recommended that people eat more whole grains and cut down on fat and cholesterol. That push for more wheat in the diet began the sharp rise in obesity.

## Growing Poverty

It's taken a number of years to recover from the Great Recession, which plunged many people into poverty (from 2008 to 2013, the number of people in America who could qualify for food stamps went from seventeen million to forty-seven million).[8] Eating healthy food on a tight budget can be a real challenge, especially considering how inexpensive processed foods have become. However, I have found in my practice that obesity crosses economic boundaries: even wealthy people eat junk food!

## Lack of Healthy Food

In some cities of the country, usually in impoverished neighborhoods, often known as food deserts, stores that sell fresh fruits and vegetables are scarce. It's easier to pick up something in a can, box, or even out of a freezer at a corner gas station than to go to a grocery store or farmer's market.[9]

## The Time Factor

When times are tough, people often work two jobs just to make ends meet. That takes away from time in the kitchen, and with family.

That poor work-life balance often leads to obesity. In 2013, the USA ranked twenty-eighth in work-life balance among the world's advanced nations.[10]

## Lack of Safe Places to Play and Exercise

In some areas of the country, it's easy to get around on foot, while in other areas a car is pretty much a necessity. The lack of a safe place to walk or jog, or for kids to play, makes getting regular exercise more challenging.

## More Stress

People often overeat when they are stressed, which can lead to weight gain.

## Lack of Sleep

In the 1960s, 8.5 hours of sleep per night was common; today, it's more like seven hours on average. Lack of sleep has consequences beyond feeling tired. Studies have found a connection between unhealthy snack cravings and larger appetites in people who don't get enough sleep.[11]

## A Changing Microbiome (Gut Chemistry)

A diet void of plant-based foods, the stress of a hectic life, more screen time, less family togetherness, an underutilization of energy, more calories taken in than burned—all these factors are changing the chemistry of the human body, creating a perfect storm for developing obesity.

Perhaps the greatest change is inside the gut. The intestinal microbiome is essentially the microorganisms in the human gut—about

100 trillion of them. They are responsible for extracting calories from food and turning them into energy. Obesity can change the ability of these microorganisms to do their job.[12] In fact, when corrupted, they can even reverse their role and add to the obesity problem while causing damaging inflammation throughout the body.

Recent research has shown that the composition of these gut bacteria is different in obese and lean individuals. It seems that the ratio of bacteroidetes and firmicutes, the two dominant intestinal bacterial in obese individuals, showed a decrease in bacteroidetes and a corresponding increase in firmicutes. This delicate balance of not only the amount of bacteria, but the corresponding ratios is of increasing importance in obesity. Fascinating research has shown that the transplant of stool (not a cheerful image) and their beneficial bacteria from a lean individual into an obese one results in weight loss.[13] Diets richer in plants, grains, and fiber promote the increase in the beneficial bacteria, altering inflammation, and increasing the beneficial byproducts of metabolism. Understanding the role of the gut microbiome in disease is far from fully understood. The early data is intriguing, but further research is required.

Part of the problem may be coming from the antibiotics and probiotics used to beef up the animals people eat. Those additives may modify the animal's gut flora, which can then corrupt the good bacteria in a person's gut and eliminate its ability to turn sugar and starch into beneficial glucose. That glucose is the energy your body uses and also stores for later, when you need it. Modified food also affects insulin, which is needed to convert the glucose to energy. So instead of having all the mechanisms in place to eat food and be powered by it, the food itself is turning into fat stores. The result? Weight gain, obesity, fatty livers, and chronic problems.

Areas of the world that don't have food additives tend to be healthier. A study of the Hadza, a tribe of hunter-gatherers in Tanzania, found that their diet of wild berries, root plants, wild meat, and honey, meant they had a greater variety of gut microbes, including helpful bacteria that are now missing from the guts of Americans.[14] The standard American diet is indeed sad.

So while obesity is the leading culprit of metabolic syndrome, other "characters" also play key roles.

## Diabetes: There's No Such Thing as Just "a Touch"

Patients often come to me with varying levels of abnormal blood sugar. It's "a touch of diabetes" they've been told by their primary care physician. When I ask the patients whether they are concerned, they usually answer, "No, because my doctor isn't." They haven't been alerted to the dangers that elevated blood sugar represents, nor have they been educated on lifestyle changes they could make to avoid problems down the road. You, as the patient, the consumer, the owner of your body, have to realize the significance these blood sugar elevations represent.

There's no such thing as "a touch of diabetes." Especially if obesity, or any of the other metabolic syndrome characters—high cholesterol, high blood pressure, NAFL—are already problems, diabetes is nothing to be taken lightly. Diabetes is a disease where the body doesn't produce enough insulin, or doesn't properly use the insulin it makes. Insulin helps convert sugars and starches to glucose to fuel the body.

Every year, some 3.2 million deaths can be attributed to complications associated with diabetes.[15] According to the American Diabetes Association, in 2015:

✓ Diabetes was the seventh leading cause of death in the USA. That figure may be underreported, since diabetes is often not listed as a cause or contributor of death in individuals who have it.

✓ 30.3 million Americans (9.4 percent of the population) had diabetes.

✓ Some 7.2 million were undiagnosed.

✓ Annually, there are 1.5 million new cases of diabetes in Americans.[16]

So "a touch of diabetes" is actually a serious condition known as prediabetes. In 2015, some 84.1 million American adults had prediabetes condition in which blood glucose levels are higher than normal but are not high enough for a diagnosis of diabetes. People with prediabetes are at increased risk for developing type 2 diabetes and for heart disease and stroke. Other names for prediabetes are impaired glucose tolerance and impaired fasting glucose.[17] Prediabetes means blood sugar levels are higher than normal, and without lifestyle changes, you're on the road to having type 2 diabetes.

Type 1 diabetes is usually diagnosed early in life, in children and young adults, earning it the name of juvenile diabetes. Only 5 percent of people with diabetes have this form of the disease. Type 1 occurs when the pancreas fails to produce insulin. It is believed that the person's own immune system destroys the insulin-producing cells in the pancreas, leading to this insulin deficiency. Maybe you or someone you know takes insulin injections every day? That's what happens with type 1 diabetes. Approximately 1.25 million American children and adults have type 1 diabetes.

Type 2 diabetes occurs when the body resists insulin (called insulin resistance). That causes blood sugar to rise, a condition known as hyperglycemia. When that happens, the pancreas tries to overcompensate by cranking out too much insulin in an attempt to stabilize blood sugar. That's a lot of wear and tear on the pancreas over time. High insulin levels also throw off the metabolism, making the body less efficient at using energy.

More than 80 percent of people with type 2 diabetes are also obese. In fact, type 2 often occurs as a result of the weight people typically gain with age. The good news is that type 2 diabetes can be managed—or even reversed—by maintaining a healthy weight, losing excess weight, and getting regular exercise.

However, type 2 diabetes also increases the risk of developing cardiovascular disease. Since it's estimated that the number of people with diabetes will double by 2025, then an increase in the number of people with cardiovascular disease is also likely.[18] That brings us to the next metabolic syndrome character, cardiovascular disease.

## Cardiovascular Disease

Cardiovascular disease affects the heart and blood vessels, usually because of a condition known as atherosclerosis, which is when the arteries that supply the heart get a buildup of plaque on the inside. Chances are you know someone who has had a heart attack or stroke—plaque buildup may be why.

Often, plaque buildup happens because of obesity. Obesity triggers abnormal changes in what are known as lipids, which are building blocks of cholesterol. There are two kinds of cholesterol in the bloodstream: low-density lipoprotein (LDL), also known as the bad cholesterol, and high-density lipoprotein (HDL), also known as the good cholesterol. The body naturally produces cholesterol, but too much of the wrong kind of cholesterol can be a bad thing because it can build up in the arteries, as plaque does. A lifestyle of eating too much unhealthy food and getting too little exercise can raise the levels of LDL and lower HDL, increasing the risk for heart disease.

Unhealthy living can also raise triglycerides, a fat in the bloodstream. When cholesterol forms in the liver, it brings triglycerides along for the ride through the bloodstream. Normally, triglycerides energize the body, but too much can raise the risk of heart disease, as too much bad cholesterol does.

Sometimes, high cholesterol just runs in the family. But most of the time, unhealthy living is the cause. The Centers for Disease Control and Prevention (CDC) estimates that 71 million American adults have high levels of low-density lipoprotein (LDL), and only one-third of them have the condition under control. As was the case with Laura, sometimes when people's liver tests show a problem, they are taken off their cholesterol-lowering statin. But again, there's no data to suggest that there's an increased risk of drug-related liver injury by taking a statin despite a constant flood of commercials alerting the public to the dangers.

Body weight can also directly affect cardiovascular risk. A higher than normal body mass index (BMI), which is a measure of body fat based on a person's height and weight, can raise blood pressure, triglycerides, blood sugar and bad cholesterol levels, and inflammation in the body. Any or all of these can increase the risk for coronary heart disease, stroke, and death.[19]

People who have too much weight around their midsection are at a greater risk for high blood pressure. According to the American Heart Association and the National Heart, Lung and Blood Institute, a woman's waist should not exceed thirty-five inches, and a man's waist shouldn't be more than forty inches. Another way to measure risk is with the waist-to-hip ratio (waist measurement divided by hip measurement). For example, a person with thirty-nine-inch hips and a thirty-inch waist would have a waist-to-hip ratio of 0.77. A healthy result should be no more than 0.85 for women and 0.90 for men.

Cardiovascular disease also increases the risk for stroke because of clogs in the arteries, or when some of that plaque breaks loose and travels to the brain.

As you can see, the diseases can build on each other; one leads to the other, to the other, to the other, and finally, to the last key character in metabolic syndrome: fatty liver.

## Your Fatty Liver

Fatty liver affects one of the most crucial organs in the body. Fatty liver is so integral to metabolic syndrome that I've devoted an entire chapter to it (chapter three). For now, let me simply define the two types of fatty liver.

NAFL means there is fat in the liver, but not much in the way of inflammation and scar tissue. NAFL is a less severe form. Still, like the other characters of metabolic syndrome, fatty liver is a red flag signaling that it's time for you to *act now* to make some changes for your body. Being told you have a fatty liver may be the earliest indicator that there is serious trouble ahead.

The more severe form is nonalcoholic steatohepatitis (NASH). NASH puts a person at risk for much more aggressive diseases since it involves inflammation and fibrosis (scar tissue) in the liver, ultimately leading to cirrhosis and even to liver cancer.

A quick side note on hepatitis: As I describe later on, hepatitis simply means inflammation of the liver. There are numerous causes for this, but in the discussion of fatty liver, *steato-hepatitis* is inflammation (or hepatitis) due to fat in the liver.

My job as a hepatologist is to determine which category you fit into, and that involves a workup of imaging, blood tests, and maybe even a liver biopsy. Fatty liver remains a major public health concern that should not to be overlooked, because of the growing number of cases of cirrhosis, liver cancer, and liver failure cases attributed to it.

Now, let's look at a few of the other characters that sometimes come with obesity and metabolic syndrome.

## Gastroesophageal Reflux Disease

There is compelling and indisputable evidence of the link between obesity, gastroesophageal reflux disease (GERD) and heartburn, and cancer of the esophagus.[20] Heartburn is the feeling or sensation of burning in the chest related to acid from the stomach irritating the esophagus, caused by GERD. GERD is the abnormal condition where acid from the stomach refluxes back from the stomach to esophagus, setting you up for damage and complications. Between 1975 and 2001, there was a sixfold increase in esophageal cancer.[21] Research is beginning to point to fatty food consumption for an increase in the number of people suffering from GERD. Chronic GERD leads to a condition called Barrett's esophagus, a premalignant condition of the mucosa of the esophagus, putting individuals with it at risk for esophageal cancer. The increase in the number of GERD cases is directly tied to the increase in obesity. Don't simply think that taking the "purple pill" is the fix for your heartburn. Weight loss and dietary improvement is the true intervention required. What else does eating fatty food lead to? Obesity, of course.

## Obstructive Sleep Apnea

Obstructive sleep apnea (OSA) is the most severe form of sleep-disordered breathing, or disruptions in breathing when a person sleeps. OSA is caused by an obstruction in the airway; in obese patients, that obstruction comes from extra fat in the throat, which can cause pressure, leading the airway to collapse at night during sleep.

If you or someone you know snores and wakes up gasping for breath, chances are that OSA is the culprit. Obese people are especially at risk. It's estimated that 25 to 45 percent of obese people have OSA.[22] And OSA isn't just an adult disease. Nearly half (46 percent) of obese children may also have it.[23]

A person carrying extra weight around the chest may also struggle to breathe. The more body fat around the chest, the more pressure there is on the lungs, and the less ability to catch a decent breath.[24]

OSA also raises the risk for high blood pressure, congestive heart failure, atrial fibrillation, insulin resistance, inflammation, and obesity—those other metabolic syndrome characters.

## Reproductive Health and the ED Connection

Being overweight also has adverse effects on the ability of a man or woman to reproduce. In women, obesity can lead to irregular cycles, miscarriages, less ability to conceive even with medical intervention, illness during pregnancy, preterm deliveries, and more complications with newborns.[25]

In men, obesity can impair hormones, reduce sperm count, and even damage sperm DNA.[26] It also plays a significant role in erectile dysfunction (ED), which is caused by decreased blood flow to the penis, and obesity affects the health of blood vessels (fatty foods and a sedate lifestyle contribute to artery narrowing and hardening). In fact, ED may be the first sign of cardiovascular disease or diabetes (obesity related), as well as hormonal changes, such as lower levels of testosterone, which is common in obese men. Instead of reaching for Viagra or Cialis, men with ED need to take stock of their weight and nutritional status. I view ED as an early warning sign for serious troubles elsewhere in your body, not just trouble in the bedroom. The manufacturers of these erectile dysfunction medications have not served the public well by refusing to alert men to the direct connection between metabolic syndrome and sexual dysfunction.

## The Cancer Link

The link between obesity and cancer is getting a lot more attention these days, and few body systems are unaffected. Multiple studies have found convincing evidence of the association between obesity and cancers of the esophagus, kidneys, liver, pancreas, colon, rectum, breast, endometrium, and gallbladder.[27]

The culprit is inflammation, which corrupts the body's tissues. Healthy cells can usually repair themselves, but when inflammation is present, those same cells may actually promote the growth and spread of cancer.[28] Processed foods, especially deli meats, salami, and hot dogs, as well as grilled beef and chicken, are the focus of intense scrutiny regarding the food-obesity-cancer connection.

## And Then There's Depression

When people have all the physical characters of metabolic syndrome—obesity, diabetes or insulin resistance, cardiovascular disease, NAFL, and others—it stands to reason they may struggle with depression. On top of the social and cultural prejudices obese people face, body chemistry changes can bring about some unwelcome feelings.[29]

Like the other metabolic syndrome characters, depression doesn't discriminate by age; it affects adults and children. Obesity and depression can be a particularly vicious coupling. When people are overweight, they may drown their sorrows by binge-eating more sweets, comfort foods, and carbohydrates, being less active while "hiding" from the world, and losing more sleep over their situation.[30] Poor body image and social stigmatization fuels poor eating habits. That's just adding to the weight, and ultimately, to the depression.

## The Cost of Obesity—Everyone is Effected

Feeling unwell makes people less productive, affects their ability to make an income, and makes it tougher to enjoy life. In short, it sucks being sick. But being sick with the diseases that comprise metabolic syndrome affects more than just the person who is sick; it affects us all.

Metabolic syndrome is a fast-growing public health issue facing our entire nation and the world. With obesity alone, healthcare costs are expected to reach $344 billion in 2018; that's projected to be $1,425 per person rising from $361 per adult as I write this book. [31]

**Here's a snapshot of what has happened across the US since 2008:**

### Rates of Obesity

|             | 2008  | 2013  | 2015  |
| ----------- | ----- | ----- | ----- |
| Mississippi | 37.7% | 44.2% | 52.2% |
| New York    | 29.4% | 34.3% | 40.2% |
| Texas       | 34.0% | 38.1% | 42.4% |

### Healthcare Spending Related to Obesity ($/Adult)

|             | 2008  | 2013  | 2015       |
| ----------- | ----- | ----- | ---------- |
| Mississippi | $441  | $738  | $1,757     |
| New York    | $341  | $568  | $1,348     |
| Texas       | $348  | $557  | $1,255[32] |

Globally, in 2014, the economic impact of obesity was estimated at $2 trillion, or 2.8 percent of the global gross domestic product.[33] Besides all the extra healthcare expenses, obesity also causes lost work days, lower work productivity, and even permanent disability. Obese male employees miss 2.5 working days more than the normal-weight male employees, and obese females miss five days more than normal-weight female employees.[34] In fact, only 3 percent of employed people account for 21 percent of obesity-related absenteeism costs.[35] That complicates employers' ability to provide affordable healthcare. How companies, both large and small, manage the health and wellness of their employees is an important discussion they are going to have to face. As the number of obese employees increases, simply as a function of the workforce demographics, strategies to keep them healthy will become important. Ignoring this will not be an option if the employer wants a present, productive, and happy workforce.

More workers' compensation claims are filed by people who are obese, often because of costs associated with the other metabolic syndrome characters. Overall, the number of disability claims in older adults has actually gone down, but those gains will soon be wiped out by rising disability claims from other diseases caused by obesity.[36] Basically, we won a war on one front, but we're being attacked on another—obesity.

Emergency room costs also take a hit. The ER costs for an obese person are 22 percent higher and for a severely obese person, 41 percent higher than for a patient of healthy weight.[37] Even moderately obese people—those with a BMI between 30 to 35—are more than twice as likely as healthy-weight individuals to be prescribed medication to manage a health problem.[38]

**Other costs related to obesity:**

- ✓ Bariatric surgery costs $14,000 to $20,000 per person, but an obese patient racks up $200,000 more in medical costs throughout that patient's lifetime.

- ✓ Obese patients do not respond well to vaccines, leaving them more susceptible to flu that can be passed along to others.

- ✓ Military recruiters often struggle to find soldiers fit enough for duty.[39]

Diabetes is also taking a toll. On average, diabetics cost the healthcare system triple what a healthy person would cost, and that doesn't include lost productivity, which was $69 billion in 2012.[40] According to the American Diabetes Association, the total cost of diabetes in the US in 2012 was $245 billion, including $176 billion in direct medical costs.

It's a frightening tale: The USA will not be able to afford metabolic syndrome. It's going to take an army of people in healthcare to handle what is essentially a very unhealthy population at a time when the healthcare system is already so overburdened it's about to implode. Physicians are retiring in record numbers, and the greatest medical system in the world will be severely handicapped in the decades to come unless we face obesity, and all of its downstream complications, honestly, for what it is. We are eating ourselves sick.

All that can change if people start taking responsibility for their health. It's time to recognize that metabolic syndrome affects everyone: the patients as well as their family, community, and country as a whole.

## Time to Stop

It's time to stop tiptoeing around the subject. When are you going to get as angry as me about the health of our country? Every day I see the suffering and *I am sickened by what I see*. It doesn't have to be that way anymore since these diseases are overwhelmingly preventable.

I got into this business to help people because I saw a great need for it. In 1988, the second year of my residency, I was working in an intensive care unit where a young teen arrived with liver failure and needed a transplant. It was a complicated case because no exact cause of the failure was identified. I was working in Brooklyn, New York, at a legendary hospital that was one of the largest teaching hospitals in the country: Kings County Hospital Center. Even at that great facility, there were no real authorities on liver disease, and in New

York, one of the biggest cities in the country, there were no transplant doctors willing to accept this case. I somehow was able to get an angel flight for the teen and his mom to take us to the University of Pittsburgh Medical Center to get him a liver transplant. Unfortunately, the transplant only kept him alive six more months. Still, with that dire human need, I found my niche. Later that year, I accompanied my older sister, Anne, to the University of Nebraska Medical Center (UNMC) in Omaha, where she would receive a bone marrow transplant for Hodgkin's disease. UNMC happened to be the finest training center for liver disease and transplants, and I had the opportunity to work with their team while staying with Anne. The eight weeks in Omaha, working with the finest liver specialists, was transformational. That stint solidified my desire to be a liver doctor.

Today, my absolute mission is to turn people around before they get to the point of needing a transplant. When patients come to me with fatty liver disease that is starting to progress, I've found that I am often the first physician to have a conversation with them about the other diseases and conditions that equate to metabolic syndrome. "Your weight is a problem," I have to tell them. "Your 'touch of diabetes,' your cholesterol levels, your five years of abnormal liver tests are problems. All of these have to be addressed—*now*." I have to inform them that the patients I currently care for in the intensive care unit (ICU), patients who are dying of end-stage liver disease from fatty liver, were, five years previously just where they are today. "I don't want you to follow their path," I tell them.

It can be difficult to make my point because even though the tests may show them headed for disaster, they generally feel okay at the time. That is unique to liver disease. It's a deadly disease that allows people to continue working, to continue their routine, without much of a hitch. The liver suffers in silence. However, left untreated, the odds of metabolic syndrome progressing to advanced liver failure are great. I've seen thousands of patients follow this collision course in misery, and ultimately, dying. So, what I'm trying to impress upon you, the readers of this book, is the importance of what I'm telling you.

Take heed. Let me get you on the path to wellness.

When it comes to turning metabolic syndrome around, there is much discussion about which is best: the carrot or the stick? I lean more toward the carrot (plus carrots are good for you!). My goal is to educate and enlighten you—for you to understand the problem so you can join the growing tide of interest in living a healthier life. My goal is to inspire you to better understand your situation and see the reality of it so you will begin to do something about it *now*.

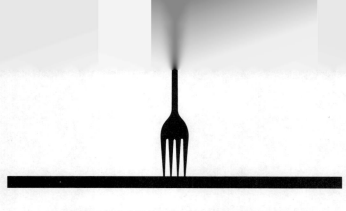

# RAISE YOUR HEALTH IQ

*Each chapter in this book ends with a series of questions you should be able to answer after reading the material I've presented. Learning this information and data is the first step in better understanding and taking the action you need to be a more informed consumer of health and wellness. If you'd like to know more about these or other topics associated with metabolic syndrome, then please visit my website at www.drjoegalati.com.*

1.  Name the conditions or diseases that comprise metabolic syndrome.

2.  How many children under age four are overweight or obese?

3.  What is the microbiome, and what role does it play in obesity?

4.  What is the most dreaded complication of nonalcoholic fatty liver disease?

5.  What condition has resulted in a sixfold increase of cancer of the esophagus?

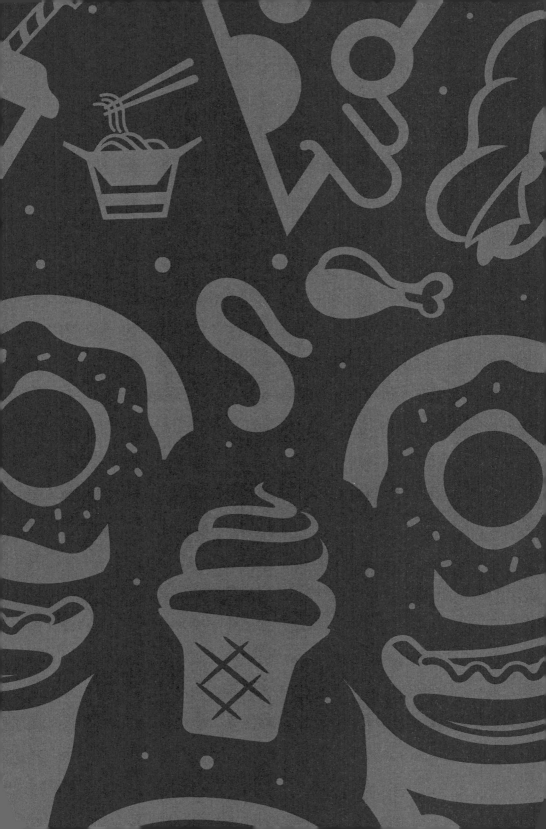

# CHAPTER 2

# The Role Of Family, Food, And Lifestyle

→ *The Fragmented Family*
→ *Home Economics: It's Not an Instinct*
→ *Confused Consumers*
→ *Too Pooped? Nonsense*
→ *No Quick-Fix Pill*

**Kathy and Chris** have been neighbors of mine for a number of years. As a result, it's given me a front-row seat into how they've raised their four children.

Over the years, in spite of their busy schedules and commitments, they've both found time to make meals a top priority. "No excuses," Kathy says when it comes to that family value.

Both are working attorneys, although Kathy stayed at home to raise the kids until their youngest started preschool. By then, the family's approach to meals was a well-oiled machine that included preparing a food list and a week's worth of menus on Sunday afternoon. Together, Kathy and Chris did the shopping and made sure the kitchen was well stocked.

On a typical day, Kathy would get up early and make a fresh breakfast for the children, which included the day's menu that had been pre-determined on Sunday. Eggs, oatmeal, cereal, fruit, or yogurt were readied as the kids prepared for school. The kids especially liked "eggs McFenelon," an egg-and-meat sandwich on half of an English muffin.

Prepping the night before also made it possible for Kathy to prepare fresh meals on weekday evenings after arriving home from work. She was able to adjust her work schedule to arrive home by 3:30 p.m. to be there for the kids after school. For fifteen years, the family followed a "Crock-Pot Wednesday" tradition. By tossing all the ingredients into the slow cooker in the morning, a delicious dinner was ready by the time the family gathered for the evening meal. "It was effortless," says Kathy.

Chris, an excellent cook in his own right, was assigned to prepare and cook every Sunday. That division of labor allowed a sense of shared responsibility for the task of feeding the family. Sundays also included a visit from Aunt Phyllis, Chris's great aunt who lived at a nearby assisted living center after relocating from New York City when she turned eighty-five. She shared stories, advice, wisdom, and even better, recipes from her Italian heritage.

Meal prep was a family activity, with the kids helping out in the kitchen by the time they were ten years old. They loved to cook and were very good at it. Now grown, the children are lean, healthy, and successful adults.

Kathy and Chris never purposely made nutrition their first priority but realized if they took an organized approach to family meals, nutrition would naturally follow. Mealtime was a cherished part of the day. They never ate out, because it was too expensive for their budget and took up too much valuable time, and they felt that food prepared at home was superior in quality and taste. As a family, they understood the importance of cooking together and breaking bread together. Today, that approach is paying dividends: a second generation is living the values of good nutrition, good health, and family togetherness.

## The Fragmented Family

Kathy and Chris's lives may seem idyllic today. Few families take the time to plan a week's worth of menus, shop for those meals, prepare ahead, and make time to sit down and eat together. Why? Largely because the family unit has become so fragmented. Today, single-parent and working-parent homes are the norm. Kids are rushed from one activity to another, getting home only in time to grab a heat-and-eat snack over homework. This is not a winning strategy.

The fragmented family unit and other changes in social structure have led to the loss of traditions such as the grandma effect, which involves regular, home-cooked meals or recipes being passed down through generations. When a grandmother is around to pass down recipes, there is often a more positive influence on having structured meals and cooking, along with other family values, as the norm. As families fragment, grandma, who used to keep the troops in line, is nowhere to be seen.

Cooking, eating healthy food, and family togetherness—these are the kinds of issues I talk with my patients about. At times, I feel as much a social scientist as I am a physician. These are the important discussions physicians need to have with their patients. The content of these conversations is as important as your doctor asking about your improvement in symptoms or how you're tolerating the latest drug therapy you were prescribed.

While a fragmented family and unhealthy eating are bad enough for adults, the impact that lifestyle is going to have on future generations is worse. Kids are being raised in environments that promote poor health. Foods loaded with sugar and lacking in nutrition are aggressively marketed to them (and to adults). Many kids' closely regimented schedules don't include time for a healthy meal. There is an entire sector of the food industry catering to the on-the-go customer. Few of these products support well-being.

The family makeup itself can increase the risk of disease. Research has shown that children in single-parent households, especially girls or an only child, are significantly more overweight or at a higher risk for obesity than kids who live with two parents and siblings. That's partly because kids left alone tend to spend more time sitting around watching TV and eating fewer meals in a family setting. They also eat fewer nutritious foods, such as fresh fruit and vegetables, instead choosing more foods high in fat and sugar. That's a problem considering the number of single-mother households in America has more than tripled since 1970, from three million then to 10 million in 2003, and single-father families also rose from less than 500,000 to more than two million.

It's unfortunate that single parents tend to have less money than two parents, and they are available less often to monitor and regulate their child's food intake and activities.

Children's health should be a top priority, regardless of the family situation. Parents worry about their kids being bullied at school, they worry about them being safe playing outside, they protect them with seat belts and helmets, and worry that they aren't being treated fairly by society. But when is there going to be the community outrage about the way kids are eating and the lack of exercise in their life? Without concern over the nutrition and exercise aspects of their life, children are being set up to become obese; they are being set up to fail from a health and wellness standpoint.

Since metabolic syndrome is going to impact everyone, the health of all children should be top of mind for everyone from teachers and coaches to caregivers and family members to frontline healthcare providers. When primary care physicians see a child of a working or single parent, they need to recognize the potential risk and raise questions to explore the issue: How are your children eating? How much time do you spend together? That is the kind of question that should be asked. My physician colleagues may reject such an approach—or request—but until we have these complex conversations, we are all complacent in perpetuating the status quo, which is not improving the health of anyone.

No parent, no caring adult would let their child ride in a car without seat belts. They wouldn't be allowed to ride off on a bike without a helmet. They wouldn't be allowed in a car with an intoxicated driver. Then why on earth are kids being allowed to eat garbage? To me, there's no difference. Picking up a burger and fries for dinner at the fast-food drive through is endangering the child. Period. Have I made my point?

# The Power of the Family Meal

It used to be that even in homes where both parents worked, morning and evening meals during the week were prepared fresh and eaten around the dining table. Anyone can discover the power of the family meal, just as Kathy and Chris did.

The power of the family meal is about nutrition—and so much more. A family that gets together regularly over a nutritious meal is going to build closer bonds that can have a tremendous windfall effect. Children who eat with their families generally have:

- ✓ healthier eating habits
- ✓ better vocabularies
- ✓ better grades
- ✓ closer family relationships
- ✓ fewer risky behaviors
- ✓ lower risk for obesity
- ✓ better overall health

Children who help prepare the food are also more likely to gain more life skills and have a greater sense of self-esteem and responsibility for themselves and others.

One of the key benefits of the family meal is that it creates a sense of structure. When everyone is responsible for showing up at a specific time and place for a meal, it adds a sense of accountability. "Dinner's at six" can become a calling, of sorts, for everyone to get together over a positive experience.

**Family mealtime is about getting back to the basics. Here are a few of my favorite tips to help make mealtime a success:**

- ✓ **Set a schedule.** As much as possible, set a regular time for everyone to get together in the kitchen for meals. If needed, start slow. Have a family night the same night each week and set aside one meal each weekend for family. If all you have is thirty minutes together three times a week, that's a start.

- ✓ **Plan ahead.** Having a plan may be the best way to ensure your family meal is a success. Set aside one day each week to plan the menu for the week and then go shopping for those meals.

- ✓ **Avoid distractions.** Turn off the TV and adopt a policy of having no cell phones at the table. That includes any electronic gadget (tablet, iPod, smartphone). One study found that American kindergartners who watched TV during dinner were more likely to be overweight by the time they were in third grade.

- ✓ **Maybe throw in a prayer.** If everyone has to sit at the table anyway, consider starting off with a prayer or even a simple round of describing what they were blessed with that day.

An added bonus of eating at home is that it saves money. Only one generation ago, more than 75 percent of the family food budget was spent on ingredients that were cooked at home. Today, more than 50 percent of food money is spent eating out. Dinner for a family of four, including four appetizers, four entrées, and three desserts, will run about $85. Think about the multiple nutritious meals you could prepare with those dollars.[41]

# Home Economics: It's Not a Natural Instinct

The remedy as I see it, again, is to get back to the basics. In spite of the fact that there are countless websites, cookbooks, TV shows, and even entire television networks dedicated to cooking, nearly a third of Americans (28 percent) still don't know how to cook properly. Millennials, especially, just don't have the skill level to cook for themselves, current research suggests.[42] They may not have been taught. They view cooking as a highly time-consuming, labor-intensive problem. They don't want to clean up afterward. So, for them, it's just easier to eat out. Patients of mine regularly complain about how much they dislike cooking because of the required kitchen cleanup afterward. I just sit there in disbelief. They are, in a sense, turning over the keys to their health and wellness and nutritional livelihood to somebody else. But once the responsibility for preparing food has been turned over, there's no telling what's being served up through a drive-through window or on a restaurant plate. Usually, it's a meal loaded with fat, sugar, salt—and excess calories. Along with that comes obesity and then all those associated diseases, aka *the other MS*.

Perhaps what's missing is a class that used to be taught for many years in schools: home economics. In the absence of a formal family structure, one way to learn the life skills needed is through the reintroduction of home economics in schools.

The home economics movement dates back to the mid-1800s, when there was a push to allow women to pursue higher education. Originally known as domestic economy, after a book written by Catherine E. Beecher, the subjects taught encompassed everything from cooking and sewing to meal planning to home management to nutrition and even dealing with family and social issues. Once the movement took hold, home economics grew until it was a course offered by nearly every school system. The courses inspired many youth to become homemakers, parents, and professionals in the food, hospitality, textiles, clothing, and interior design industries.

Over time, however, the teaching of home economics in schools waned due to a number of factors, including the belief that an understanding of domestic matters was not a subject requiring a formal education, as if humans should just instinctively know how to cook, clean, and manage a home. Interestingly, my daughter (who likes to cook) is something of a kitchen guru among her college friends, many of whom, literally, don't even know how to boil water. How sad!

That really comes as no surprise, considering many young people have never learned basic life skills. What does it say about our culture when we have an entire generation that is disconnected from the kitchen? What was so important for parents fifteen or twenty years ago that they never taught their kids the skills they would need to leave home and thrive? We are now faced with an entire generation that is simply not interested in the preparation of food, nutrition, and the impact food has on their well-being. Am I overreacting? The data suggests I am not.

What it may come down to is simply better time management. People should take a break from programming a new phone or gadget and, instead, organize a few menus, create a shopping list, go to the store, and pick up food for four or five days. Or they should delegate responsibilities to other family members and just get started figuring out what to do. Half the fun of a family cooking and eating together may be in the trial and error that comes from the new adventure itself.

# Food for Convenience

One reason we're where we are today is because of the rise of convenience and processed foods. The problem is that such foods have helped create an obese-promoting environment.

It used to be that eating out was something done to celebrate a special event; it wasn't a daily habit. Now, a home-cooked meal is the exception rather than the rule in America. With the erosion of the family unit, any meals that are eaten at home take only minutes to prepare because so many foods are heat-and-eat, loaded with preservatives and other unhealthy and non-nutritious ingredients. Ready-made food lacking in significant nutrition is available everywhere you look. Drive-through, fast-food restaurants line roadways. Supermarkets have more than their share of unhealthy food to-go. For a snack, there's the local vending machine or corner quick stop. For lunch, there's fast food across the street from work.

In fact, studies of Americans found that

- as much as 20 percent of all meals are eaten in the car;

- as a nation, we consume 31 percent more packaged than fresh food;

- more than half (52 percent) of the population believe doing their taxes is easier than understanding good nutrition;

- at least one-fourth of the population eat fast food daily.[43]

As people turn to fast foods for convenience, major supermarket chains are responding with increasing availability of ready-to-go meals. They know what consumers want, but is this right? There are entire sections of the grocery store dedicated to letting you walk in and pluck something off the shelf that you can eat while walking to the car if you want to. It may be something freshly prepared at the store, but it's still, essentially, today's version of a frozen dinner, something loaded with fat, sugar, salt, and calories. Oh, and by the way, they're also costlier, an added expense of letting someone else do the work you could do.

In fact, only 10 percent of items sold in supermarkets are fresh produce, while 15 percent are dairy and frozen foods, and half are the items sold in aisles or from displays.[44] Millennials are actually driving an increase in grocery stores that provide these ready-made meals, called *grocerants*. More than three-quarters of millennials purchase items from grocerant stores at least once a month. And it's a trend that's catching on with others: more than 65 percent of generation Xers and 60 percent of baby boomers report they have also bought food from such stores at least once a month.[45]

## Confused Consumers

Today, the number of products for consumers to choose from in a grocery store is staggering. One group estimates that the number of products on store shelves swelled between 1975 and 2008 from around 8,900 to nearly 47,000. Do we really need that many items to select from? According to the USDA, the number of new food and beverage products on store shelves reached a new high in 2016, with the top items on the list being beverages, snacks, bakery foods, sauces, condiments, and dressings.

All those choices lead to consumer confusion. We used to be able to look for plain old Quaker Oats oatmeal—no preservatives, no fat, no sugar. Now there are fifteen different kinds of oatmeal: instant, one-minute, three-minute, five-minute, and every flavor in the world. It's enough to make consumers throw up their hands and head over to the local McDonald's for an Egg McMuffin.

I see that confusion every day with my patients. They don't know what food to buy. Even when they try to find something they believe is healthy, they quickly become overwhelmed by the choice. They find the grocery shelf containing oatmeal and they believe oatmeal is oatmeal. Unfortunately, some of those oatmeal varieties are loaded with chemicals, flavorings, and all kinds of bad-for-you stuff. And where's the plain old good-for-you Quaker Oats? On the top shelf, above eye level.

Amid all the confusion are advertisers bombarding consumers with all sorts of health claims. A lot of junk food is disguised as healthy food; the labels claim the items are low in fat, calories, and sodium. Patients are always bringing me pictures of food or Internet print-outs to ask me if the item is a healthy choice, and I have to advise them they've been duped and shouldn't buy such garbage. They think, because the package has a little red heart on it, the American Heart Association has, in a sense, approved the food and it's good for them. What they don't realize is that in some instances, the serving size is very small. Many frozen dinners contain two servings, but the consumer may think the whole dinner is just one serving. This misunderstanding results in a doubling of calories, salt, and fat. Just because an Oreo is "fat-free" and has less than 100 calories, it doesn't mean a whole bag should be eaten in one or two sittings. Yes, people are thinking like that—and doing it.

There's also a lack of understanding of the ingredients in processed foods. A product that claims to be fat-free may be loaded with salt or sugar to make it taste better in the absence of what actually could have been a healthy fat. Perfectly healthy foods are being processed into something that is unhealthy. Speaking of fats, there are healthy fats to consider eating. Omega-3 and omega-6 fatty acids are beneficial, and need to be included in our diets. Obtained from fish, nuts, and seeds, more omega-3 fatty acids should be consumed. Monosaturated and polyunsaturated fats from avocados, olives and olive oil, and medium chain triglycerides found in coconut oil need to be regular staples of your diet.

Processed foods are foods that have been manufactured, or treated in some way to help them retain their shelf life. All the good components are stripped out and replaced with undesirable ingredients.

This engineering of food is done so that it will, basically, melt in your mouth. Food makers don't want you to chew too much, and they engineer food to discourage you from doing so. From a marketing standpoint, too much chewing is bad. How lazy have we all gotten? They want you to enjoy what you're eating so you'll eat more. In fact, many processed foods are actually engineered with chemicals to be hyperflavored so that biting into them makes you want more. The flavors explode in your mouth. Just a bit of chewing, and down it goes, allowing you to reach for another bite, and another … It's just that simple, and we have all fallen for these tricks at the expense of our health.

### The Problems with Processed Food

✓ **Excess sugar**. Processed food usually contains empty calories, which may taste good but have no nutritional value. Sugar can also impact your metabolism, leading to insulin resistance, elevated triglycerides and bad cholesterol, and more fat in the liver. Sound familiar?

✓ **Excess salt (sodium):** Thanks to its chemical nature, salt has the amazing ability to intensify agreeable tastes and diminish disagreeable ones. Humans like salt, but processed foods are inexcusably high in sodium content. Natural foods do not have sodium levels to be concerned about. Excess sodium leads to weight gain and fluid retention (edema), and increased blood pressure. The daily limit of sodium should be around 1,500 mg for the entire day. The standard American diet supplies you with over 3,000 mg daily. Please note: the Marie Callender's brand of beef pot pie serves 660 mg of sodium per serving (Please note a serving is half a pot pie. Who eats half a pot pie? Remember serving size I discussed previously?). It is impossible to maintain a low sodium diet while eating out or eating processed foods.

✓ **Addictive by design**. Eating too much sugar can also screw up your brain. Processed foods are designed to make you want more—and even become addictive—by appealing to the reward center of the brain. They do that by stimulating the neurotransmitter dopamine (a feel-good brain chemical) because they are engineered to work around your body's natural ability to defend itself against unhealthy energy sources. So there's science behind that nagging sweet tooth. In fact, studies have found that foods high in sugar or fat work just as addictive narcotics do. The same drug prescribed for opioid addiction can also help people lose weight.

✓ **Low nutritional value**. Even when a label appears to indicate the food is healthy, having a long list of vitamins and minerals your body needs, those ingredients may be synthetic chemical additives rather than naturally occurring nutrients.

✓ **Too easy to eat**. Processing also removes fiber, which is good for you, helping you feel full more quickly. Since they are made easier to eat, again by design, processed foods require less energy to consume and digest.

Once patients begin to understand how processed food labeling can be so deceptive, they often ask me whether the food manufacturers are purposely trying to fool people. That can certainly be the intent of labeling. Ever seen a bottle of water with "gluten-free" on the label? Well, of course bottled water is gluten-free; there's no wheat in water. It's the same with most potato chips and corn chips. Potatoes and corn don't contain gluten; they never did. But that doesn't mean the chips in that bag aren't loaded with fat, salt, calories, and unhealthy preservatives and additives.

The research suggests there are thousands of healthy products that food companies could sell. Instead, they supply unhealthy foods people really don't need, and they add to the confusion with all kinds of eye-catching, taste-bud-appealing advertising to persuade the already confused consumer to reach for something just because it's labeled "new."

Food industry marketers know the power of the buying impulse. They get that your day is hectic and you're stressed. Remember the slogan "You deserve a break today?" Fixing breakfast, lunch, and dinner— that's what they want you to break from. Some of my patients are buying it: they eat out nearly every meal.

Learning to eat better starts by understanding all the bull you're being fed. In the chapters ahead, I'll get into more details to help you become a better consumer of health, wellness, and nutrition.

For starters, many people have a false belief that natural, unprocessed food is too expensive to eat. All it takes is a little homework to figure out that that is not true. When you plan ahead, you can find deals on foods or even buy in bulk. Farmers' markets also sell locally grown, relatively inexpensive fruits and vegetables. How much can you save by buying a bag of onions or apples instead of a few out of a bin? How much saving comes from buying eighteen eggs instead of a dozen? How much can you save by buying a whole chicken and roasting it for your family of four, instead of buying a bucket of fried chicken? It may seem only a few dollars or cents here or there, but all those pennies can add up to savings, especially in the form of better overall health.

## Too Pooped? Nonsense

Back in 1950, fitness guru Jack Lalanne talked about Americans suffering from what he called "pooped-out-itis." I was lucky enough to get him as a guest on my radio show before he passed away at age ninety-six in 2011, and he was still just as amazing as he was back when he was all the rage. He told my listeners they could not succumb to being pooped out. They could not sit at home and not cook and not exercise. If they were to eat nutritious, natural foods, they would gain vitality.

Even when he was at the height of his popularity, in the 1950s and 1960s, he had segments on his television fitness show about cooking a wholesome meal. At the time, he was already raising the alarm to steer clear of processed, convenience foods. He touted eating fresh fish, meat, and vegetables. He must have been doing something right because to celebrate his seventieth birthday, he swam 1.5 miles while towing seventy boats and seventy people, all while handcuffed and shackled.

Too many people today have the false sense that they're too busy. As a result, they're eating without giving it any thought. Eat breakfast. Check. Eat lunch. Check. Eat dinner. Check. They're checking the boxes, but they don't know what's in the boxes. The idea that there's no time to cook, no time to eat healthy food, is ill-conceived.

I like to think I'm a busy guy. I'm up at five in the morning, and I work long days. All day, every day, I answer calls from patients. I don't get home some nights until after nine, but even then, it's not unusual for me to be chopping up vegetables to roast or grill, or putting together a soup, all in an effort to have food prepared for the next few days.

If I can do it, I know you can as well. I know you can find ways to make healthier food choices during the day. I know you can figure out a way to carve out twenty minutes a day to go shopping or to prepare food or to get in a bit of exercise.

Again, why am I telling you this? Because I see such a huge problem. Liver disease is a dreadful situation. Today, there are pacemakers and defibrillators for failing hearts, dialysis for failing kidneys, respirators for failing lungs, and artificial knees, hips, shoulders, and wrists. But there is still no artificial liver that can be implanted. A lot of young people, middle-aged people, and older adults are dying from liver disease, and I am witness to not only the personal pain and suffering of these patients but also to what their families endure during and after.

Most of the time, it comes down to lifestyle decisions made five or ten years earlier. I realize that if I succeed in getting the message out about metabolic syndrome, I risk putting myself out of business—and I can think of no better reason for doing so.

Healthier lifestyle choices have to be made if we're going to turn around metabolic syndrome and its devastating elements. That means getting away from a sedentary lifestyle. In a world of electronics, people sit at their desk in front of a computer all day, and then go home and sit in front of the TV. Everyone has one or more electronic gadgets that encourage more sitting and playing, viewing, or tapping out a conversation. Few people get the exercise they need and there's no denying the link between obesity and TV watching. Kids don't play outside out of concern for their safety. After work, people sit down in an easy chair and snack on whatever's available. It's late, so they don't exercise and then they head off to bed where they suffer from acid reflux and sleep apnea, both of which are obesity-related conditions. They wake up tired and go to work, grabbing a fast-food breakfast taco along the way. They eat junk for lunch. And the cycle goes on and on for days and years at a time. I listen to this same scenario every day from my patients, so I am confident in sharing this with you that this is not an isolated event experienced by a few individuals.

Somewhere along the line, there are opportunities to break the cycle. There's an old saying: "Eat breakfast like a king, lunch like a prince, and dinner like a pauper." If you don't adopt that mindset, you're headed for a vicious cycle of illness, a vicious cycle of feeling like crap.

## No Quick-Fix Pill

Almost daily, I have to explain to patients that they have chronic liver disease due to their obesity and they have all the other diseases that comprise metabolic syndrome. Sometimes, in going over their tests, I have to explain they are at increased risk for more complicating factors such as cirrhosis or liver cancer or even progressive liver failure and that they will need a liver transplant.

We outline the plan of attack—better nutrition, weight loss, exercise, getting their diabetes and blood pressure under better control, possible research study participation, and my working in concert with either their primary care physician or other doctors to help all that happen. I spend a lot of time giving them resources, educating them, and getting them more comfortable to ask the questions they want answers for. I want to empower them to understand the full scope of the problem, how we are going to work as a team, and their responsibilities.

When the consultation is finished, I ask: "Do you have any additional questions?" Invariably, they want to know, "Will I get a prescription for any of this?" To which I reply, "Yes, I'm prescribing broccoli four times a week." They smile with some reservation on their face. Broccoli, really? I tell my patients that short of me and my team heading to their home to cook dinner for them, they are going to have to decide if now is the time to make changes in how they view their health, in deciding if they want to spend the next (or last) five years of their life suffering, in how they shop, cook, and where they eat—at home, rather than at a restaurant or drive-through window.

Although they may be starting to understand their situation, they still don't really grasp its severity. They don't understand their disease may seem like clouds on the horizon now, but it's going to whip up a gale and come blow the roof off their life if they don't make changes. Many of them are justifiably concerned about their ability to turn things around in time. But a pill is not the answer.

The truth is that there is no pill, no herbal supplement, no medicine that is going to reverse metabolic syndrome on its own without significant—and permanent—lifestyle changes. In the next chapter, I think you'll get a much better understanding of what I mean.

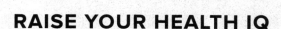

# RAISE YOUR HEALTH IQ

*Remember that healthy eating and family meals are the best ways to turn around metabolic syndrome.*

*If you'd like to know more about these or other topics associated with family meals and better nutrition, please visit my website at www.drjoegalati.com.*

1. Children of single-parent families are at risk for what health complication?

2. What benefits might children experience if their family regularly eats meals together?

3. What percentage of meals do Americans consume in their cars?

4. Between 1975 and 2008, how many additional products have become available on supermarket shelves in America?

5. True or false: Natural and unprocessed foods are more expensive than processed food?

# CHAPTER 3

# Fatty Liver Disease: The Ugly Truth

→ *The Complex Liver*
→ *Misconceptions about Liver Disease*
→ *Liver Disease: A Heartbreaking Illness*
→ *Who's Going to Provide Care?*
→ *There Is Hope*

**Meg was a** fifty-eight-year old executive who went to see her doctor because of pain in the right side of her abdomen, just below her rib cage. Ultimately, she had to have her gallbladder removed and, during the surgery, the surgeon saw that her liver was also diseased. Meg had cirrhosis. Cirrhosis happens as a result of long-term damage to the liver, when scar tissue replaces healthy liver tissue. A biopsy of Meg's liver showed that she had a large amount of fat and scar tissue from cirrhosis.

Meg had been morbidly overweight (reminder: BMI > 40) for nearly ten years before the cirrhosis was discovered. During that time, she had occasional problems with her blood sugar, but interestingly, she had no documented diabetes or high blood pressure. So, it was a bit shocking for doctors to find her cirrhosis, and needless to say, Meg and her family were devastated by the diagnosis. That's when they came to see me for a second opinion. It was my role to tell Meg and her family that it was time to take a negative and turn it into a positive. The newly diagnosed cirrhosis put her at high risk for further complications, including the risk of developing liver cancer. Needing a liver transplant was also something she might have to face in the years to come. I shared with them the next best steps to help them turn around the entire family's nutrition and lifestyle, and they promised to go shopping on the way home and clean out all the processed foods from the cabinets, freezer, and refrigerator when they got there. After a serious conversation about a commitment to make positive changes in behavior, Meg and her family finally changed their eating habits for the better, which have persisted over time for the better.

## The Complex Liver

The liver is one of the most vital organs in the body, yet many people—including many of my patients—don't even know where the liver is in the body. Located in the right upper quadrant, just under and behind the rib cage, it is by far the most complicated organ in the body. It is involved in over two hundred vital biologic reactions, including manufacturing and synthesizing a wide range of hormones, clotting factors, cholesterol, and other proteins. Since it is such a complex organ, it has been nearly impossible to replicate. For over twenty-five years, researchers have been trying to develop an artificial liver and have never really managed to create one because of the complexity of the biochemistry that's involved.

Cirrhosis occurs when healthy, functioning liver tissues are replaced by nonfunctioning scar tissue, over time. With cirrhosis, the liver loses what is commonly known as its synthetic capability, in other words, its ability to synthesize the very proteins and hormones required for life. A liver with cirrhosis, regardless of the cause, puts you at risk for liver cancer, also called hepatocellular carcinoma. To get an idea of the difference between a healthy functioning liver and one that is riddled with cirrhosis, go to www.drjoegalati.com.

Now, it's true that the liver is capable of regenerating itself. In the very early stages of scarring, there is the potential to reverse some of the damage. But when it is subjected to a destructive, ongoing, vicious cycle of damage-regeneration-damage-regeneration, it begins to develop irreversible scar tissue. Ultimately, that leads to the development of cirrhosis. Once cirrhosis has reached more advanced stages, there's very little that can be done short of a transplant. Without a transplant, death is forthcoming.

While organ transplants have been perfected over the past thirty years, we still face challenges. Transplants in the USA are overseen by UNOS, the United Network for Organ Sharing. According to UNOS, as I write this chapter:

✓ There are 116,516 people waiting for an organ transplant. That includes all organs, not just livers. There are 26,732 patients ages thirty-five to forty-nine, and 51,758 patients, ages fifty to sixty-four, waiting for organs on this list.

✓ Nearly 31,000 transplants were performed in 2015 from just over 15,000 donors. Donors can supply more than one organ, which accounts for the number of transplants being double the number of donors.

✓ In 2016, 7,841 livers were transplanted.

- ✓ Of the more than 116,000 patients waiting for organs, 14,176 were in need of a liver.

- ✓ Every year, 15 to 25 percent of patients waiting for an organ transplant die waiting for a matching organ, mostly because they become too sick to undergo a transplant, and because donors are not readily available.

- ✓ Some potential liver organ donors themselves have fatty liver and are determined to be poor donors, further limiting potential donors. Oddly, this is another unforeseen complication of metabolic syndrome and fatty liver disease: a decreased organ donor pool.

It's time to take control of the factors leading to liver disease before it's too late. Waiting for a transplant should not be part of the treatment plan.

## Misconceptions about Liver Disease

There is a strong misconception that cirrhosis is only caused by excess alcohol consumption. When I tell patients they have cirrhosis of the liver, their first response is usually, "I don't drink. I was never an alcoholic." But excess alcohol consumption accounts for only about half (49 percent) of all cirrhosis cases. The other incidences of cirrhosis (51 percent) are related to fatty liver, hepatitis C, hepatitis B, and a host of genetic abnormalities that people are, unfortunately, born with. Cirrhosis caused by non-alcoholic fatty liver disease (NAFLD) is the number-one disease leading to liver transplant, having surpassed hepatitis C in 2016.

Cirrhosis, typically, takes years to develop. NAFLD is more common in obese people, and as many as 7 percent of normal-weight people also have NAFLD. High-calorie diets that include consumption of excess saturated fats, refined carbohydrates, and high-fructose and sugar-sweetened foods and beverages have been associated with NAFLD.[46]

Prior to the early 1990s, the teaching doctrine in medical science was that alcohol was the lone culprit for fatty liver. During training, doctors were taught that alcoholics were principally the only patients who acquired fatty liver due to certain nutritional deficiencies that developed with chronic alcohol use. During the late 1980s, increased numbers of patients started being diagnosed with fatty livers because of the advent of two technologies that allowed for more investigation of the organs in the abdomen. One of those technologies was laparoscopic surgery, which allowed for less invasive surgery in the abdomen, especially gallbladder surgery. Studies show a 22 to 57 percent increase in gallbladder surgery since the introduction of laparoscopic techniques.[47] While they were investigating the gallbladder for disease, surgeons also were looking at the liver (since the gallbladder is attached to the liver), which led to more fatty livers being suspected, leading, in turn, to more biopsies, and the discovery of more cases of fatty liver and cirrhosis. The other technology was the CAT scan, a radiology imaging technique that analyzes internal organs and can measure the amount of fat in the liver. So, between surgeons looking at the liver and doing biopsies, and radiologists documenting a fatty liver on a scan, the medical field began to be inundated with reports of people having a fatty liver.

Many years ago, once a person was diagnosed with fatty liver or cirrhosis, the first question often asked by the doctor was "How much alcohol do you drink?"

To which the patient would usually politely reply, "I don't drink," or "I don't drink much alcohol at all."

The doctor would then question whether the patient was telling the truth, "Are you sure? You must be out drinking because only alcoholics or heavy alcohol abusers get a fatty liver." It took several years to realize there is a subclass of patients who have a fatty liver that is not alcohol related, hence the term *nonalcoholic fatty liver disease* (NAFLD).

Another subclass is categorized as NAFL (without the *D* for "disease"). NAFL occurs when there is fat in the liver, but there is no inflammation or scarring. NAFLD is when there is fat and inflammation and that inflammation is what leads to significant damage from the formation of fibrosis and cirrhosis. Patients with either NAFL or NAFLD don't feel sick; they don't have symptoms. That's why it's easy to procrastinate and put off turning their lifestyle around. But sadly, that's the kind of thinking that can lead to disaster. As I have stated previously, the liver suffers in silence.

The presence of biopsy-proven NAFLD varies depending on the patient population. Worldwide, the prevalence of NAFLD is estimated at 10 to 35 percent of the population. In the USA, it's estimated that 30 to 40 percent of adults have NAFLD.[48]

Another category of liver disease, known as nonalcoholic steatohepatitis (NASH), is more aggressive. With NASH, there is a higher probability of inflammation and the development of fibrosis, cirrhosis, and liver cancer. It's estimated that NASH occurs in around 15 to

20 percent of patients who have NAFLD.[49] Generally, NASH is the most aggressive form of fatty liver.

While there is no guarantee that NAFLD will progress to NASH and/or cirrhosis, NAFLD is underdiagnosed, undertreated, and underappreciated by the medical community. Every day, patients are told they have a fatty liver, but they are dependent on their family physician or other specialist telling them exactly how serious their situation is. They often aren't told they have a chance of developing cirrhosis, and they aren't told about the lifestyle changes they need to make beyond, maybe, advice to "lose some weight." So, they don't take their situation seriously.

## Liver Disease: A Heartbreaking Illness

Even without a current diagnosis for fatty liver, you may still fit into a high-risk category for fatty liver. Again, fatty liver is the liver manifestation of metabolic syndrome. The other characters of metabolic syndrome—obesity, diabetes or insulin resistance, high cholesterol—increase the risk for fatty liver. In studies of obese patients undergoing bariatric surgery, 90 percent have NAFLD, and around 5 to 8 percent of them already have cirrhosis. Type 2 diabetes also increases the probability of having fatty liver. Studies have shown that 70 percent of people with type 2 diabetes who have gone in for an ultrasound were found to have fatty liver. And half of the people with high triglycerides and low HDL (bad cholesterol) are found to have fatty liver.

Since metabolic syndrome is an early warning of liver disease, the symptoms may not come from the liver itself but from one of the other characters: obesity, diabetes, or heart disease.

If you have any of those comorbidities, those other metabolic syndrome characters, then you are at a higher risk for the development of more scar tissue and cirrhosis, which means you're at risk for liver cancer, liver failure, and maybe, even the need for a liver transplant.

## Liver Disease Warning Signs

- ✓ **increasing fatigue**
- ✓ **increasing weight**
- ✓ **increasing edema and swelling in the legs**
- ✓ **swelling and weight gain in the abdomen (ascites)**
- ✓ **loss of upper-body muscle, or muscle wasting**
- ✓ **yellowing of the skin**
- ✓ **jaundice of the eyes**

It has become popular with the lay public to refer to liver disease as the silent killer. While I have never truly liked this characterization, probably because not every liver issue will kill you, it does have some credence because all too many patients I have cared for over the past twenty-five years arrive too late to benefit from an early diagnosis and intervention. But liver disease is called the silent killer because it often doesn't reveal any real outward signs of problems until it's too late. Unlike the gallbladder, pancreas, and other abdominal organs, fatty liver really doesn't cause pain or abdominal distress. It's easy for people to ignore it and have a false sense of security that they're well.

The first sign of a problem is often fatigue, something most people just tolerate by moping along. They make up excuses such as stress, a bad marriage, shift work, or other possible causes. But at age thirty, forty, or fifty, it's not normal to be "just tolerating" fatigue. If you're obese, fatigue may be a sign of sleep apnea. It may be related to acid reflux (GERD), which is causing an unrecognized disturbance in your sleeping pattern. Fatigue can also be an early symptom of diabetes, hormonal imbalances, anemia, or a yet-to-be-diagnosed cardiovascular disease or malignancy.

People also have a tendency to tolerate gradual weight gain. Obesity doesn't usually happen as a fifty-pound gain over six months. It's gradual, a pound or two every month adding up over several years. With so many extra pounds added on, people tend to overlook another symptom of liver problems: swelling of the legs and feet. Often, they'll just chalk it up to being on their feet too long.

With cirrhosis, healthy, functioning, metabolically active liver cells are replaced with scar tissue, which, essentially, doesn't work. Because of the scar tissue in the liver, circulation in the liver is altered and a condition known as portal hypertension develops. Complications of portal hypertension include ascites, which is a buildup of fluid in the abdomen.

| Complications Of Cirrhosis | | |
|---|---|---|
| Ascites *(fluid in the abdomen)* | Anemia *(low hemoglobin)* | Gastrointestinal bleeding |
| Muscle wasting | Thrombocytopenia *(low platelet count)* | Spontaneous bacterial peritonitis *(abdominal infection of ascites)* |
| Malnutrition | Hepatorenal syndrome *(kidney failure)* | Osteopenia and osteoporosis *(bone loss)* |
| Hepatic encephalopathy *(mental confusion state)* | Hepatopulmonary syndrome *(low blood oxygen levels)* | Splenomegaly *(spleen enlargement)* |
| Pulmonary hypertension *(elevated lung pressures)* | Esophageal varices *(varicose veins in the esophagus)* | Hepatoma *(liver cancer)* |

One of the dangers of ascites is the development of what's known as spontaneous bacterial peritonitis, which is an infection of the ascites fluid. Peritonitis is a potentially life-threatening complication. Another complication of cirrhosis and portal hypertension includes hepatic encephalopathy, which is a state of confusion due to the buildup of toxins that affect the central nervous system. Portal hypertension also increases the risk of hemorrhage, or bleeding from varicose veins that develop in the esophagus and the stomach, a condition known as esophageal or gastric varices. Each one of these complications of portal hypertension increases a person's mortality or likelihood of not surviving.

Additionally, the risk of kidney failure increases. That is a condition known as hepatorenal syndrome.

Once portal hypertension develops, it's time to be evaluated for a liver transplant. But the truth is, there currently aren't enough livers to fill the need, and in the current organ allocation system, only the very sickest individuals receive transplants.

That is determined by what is known as the MELD score, which stands for the model for end-stage liver disease. Introduced on February 27, 2002, UNOS has adopted this method to allocate donor organs. This calculation is a very accurate measure of determining the risk of dying in patients with end-stage liver disease. It is used as a disease severity index to help prioritize allocation of organs for transplant. Those with the best chance of survival without a liver transplant and the *lowest* MELD scores are considered a low priority for life-saving transplants, while those having the *highest* MELD scores are the sickest with the lowest chance of survival. The latter are given a higher priority because of their reduced chance of survival without a liver transplant. The motto of "sickest first" is currently applied to patients awaiting a liver transplant. The MELD score is calculated by taking the patient's blood values of sodium, bilirubin (a measure of liver function based on bile production), creatinine (an indicator of kidney function), and the INR (international normalized ratio) for prothrombin time, which determines the liver's blood-clotting ability). These values are plugged into a mathematical formula (there are MELD score calculators available online). The values range from 5 to 40, with the expected three-month mortality (death) rates below:

| MELD Score | Mortality Probability |
| --- | --- |
| 40 | 71.3% mortality |
| 30–39 | 52.6% mortality |
| 20–29 | 19.6% mortality |
| 10–19 | 6.0% mortality |
| 9 or less | 1.9% mortality |

Some regions of the USA only offer transplants to patients with very high MELD scores, which means they perform transplants only on the sickest of the sickest. Patients in those regions are usually critically ill, maybe on dialysis for failing kidneys, on a respirator to breathe, and may have only days or weeks to live without a liver transplant. It's a very, very high risk situation to be in.

There's no doubt that liver cancer is seen with increased frequency in patients that have NASH and cirrhosis. That usually develops when patients are in the end stages of the disease. Depending on the size and location of the cancer, these patients actually get priority for a transplant.

That is the world I live in. I work with patients in this situation every day. They often tell me things such as, "Dr. Galati, I feel terrible right now. I can't work. I can't go fishing anymore. I can't go on vacation with my family. Are you telling me that I have to get sicker than this before I can have a transplant?" The answer is yes. Every day, I have to talk with families about a loved one who is dealing with these problems.

The reality is that approximately 30 percent of my patients who are on the waiting list for liver transplants die because they become too sick for a transplant. That appears to be about the national average, according to the Organ Procurement and Transplantation Network, which reports that, between 2011 and 2014, just over 67 percent of patients waiting for a new liver actually received a transplant.[50] It's heartbreaking.

End-stage liver disease is agonizing. It is a slow, painful death. And it's painful for everyone involved, the patient, family, friends, and healthcare providers. It's tough for us to watch patients we've known for a while get as sick as they do. We want to try to save everybody, even though we know we can't. Every day, we ask ourselves how many people we could have saved if we had been able to intervene one or two years earlier. That's the part of this job that's really tough.

That's why, for the last twenty-five years, I have worked to intervene earlier in the disease process. I want to minimize the amount of time I spend standing outside the ICU waiting-room door as I console family members who wish they could turn back the clock.

## Who's Going to Provide Care?

One of my concerns about the whole situation is what I see in the healthcare industry as a whole. Currently, there are not enough formally trained liver specialists to see all the patients who have a need. Becoming a hepatologist (liver specialist) is hard work that begins with completing medical school, followed by a three-year residency training program in internal medicine, followed by a three- to four-year gastroenterology fellowship, which concentrates on diseases of the liver and disorders of the digestive tract. Usually, the dedicated liver training takes place at a hospital or medical center that is affiliated with a liver transplant program. Young physicians today tend to prefer following a path in gastroenterology, concentrating on intestinal disorders and performing endoscopic procedures, rather than tackling the needs of patients with liver disease. If this need continues to grow, what's going to happen when the fatty liver epidemic reaches estimated crisis levels in 2030?

It's crucial to work now to turn the tide. It's crucial for adults who are overweight to take a look at their lives and decide that lifestyle changes must be made. And we must look at future generations: kids in school, college-age men and women, young moms and dads. We've got to address metabolic syndrome so that younger generations today are not riddled with end-stage liver disease in their forties and fifties. It's a dreadful thought.

## There Is Hope

Yes, liver disease is an ugly picture, but there is hope.

Many of my patients are self-referred, having found my practice online at www.texasliver.com, or through my weekly radio program, *Your Health First*, which is also online at www.yourhealthfirst.com, or through social media sites. They've sought me out because they've been told there is something wrong with their liver, and a family member or friend has told them they need to look into it further.

But by the time they come to me, many have advanced scarring and fibrosis. Once someone comes to me with fatty liver or a further progression of liver disease, we have a far more detailed conversation to put their situation into perspective.

When we're able to intervene earlier, when we identify that a patient is on the road to having metabolic syndrome by being overweight and having prediabetes or high blood pressure, we don't fall back on the punch line, "Eat more fruits and vegetables." My staff and I know that simply snapping out some recommendations is an unrealistic way of turning things around. Instead, we guide patients through a detailed assessment that looks at eating patterns, snacking, family structure, barriers to exercise, barriers to eating right, and more. We ask questions such as who is living at home with you? Do you have little children? Do you work shift work? Are you a caretaker for someone with special needs? How do the dynamics of your life positively or negatively impact your ability to shop, cook, eat, and prepare food? What are the obstacles to going to the gym or going for a thirty-minute bike ride, four days a week? For many people, turning around a lifestyle begins by learning what healthy food looks like. (Hint: American Chinese food may have a lot of meat and vegetables, but most of it is still fattening and loaded with sodium.)

**We're educating patients with real-world knowledge. Want to know more? Check out the Great American Produce Giveaway at www.drjoegalati.com.**

In chapter ten, I'll discuss a little further some of the dedicated protocols, intervention strategies, education, and services that are available through the Liver Specialists of Texas and the Metabolic and Fatty Liver Center.

Liver disease is a harsh reality. Turning around fatty liver begins with education, and that begins by understanding your body.

# RAISE YOUR HEALTH IQ

*Remember that metabolic syndrome will cut your life short. Starting early to turn your lifestyle around is key.*

*If you'd like to know more about these or other ways to turn around metabolic syndrome, please visit my website at www. drjoegalati.com.*

1.  Name three functions that the liver performs.

2.  What percentage of cases of cirrhosis is related to alcohol?

3.  Name the early warning signs of advanced liver disease.

4.  Portal hypertension is a complication of what disease?

5.  Why is liver disease called the silent killer?

# CHAPTER 4

# It's Your Body: Learn How It Works

→ **Body Mass Index (BMI)**
→ **Cholesterol**
→ **Diabetes**
→ **Liver Tests**
→ **Medications: Not Always Safe**
→ **Next Steps**
→ **Listen to Your Body**

**Bob is the** fifty-three-year-old owner of a small insurance company with twenty employees. His office system consists of thirty computers networked throughout three locations. When his system was compromised by a virus, it cost him over $20,000 to have it repaired by his IT team. When they realized the problem was out-of-date virus protection, he ostracized Bob, saying, "None of this would have happened if you had kept your antivirus protection up-to-date."

When Bob's business was jeopardized, he quickly shelled out tens of thousands of dollars to get it back up and running and protect it from future harm. Meanwhile, Bob is failing to protect himself against serious illness. He eats poorly, doesn't exercise, and doesn't get regular vaccinations. As a result, he is overweight, out of shape, has prediabetes, has high blood pressure, and isn't protected against influenza, hepatitis A and B, and other preventable diseases. And it's going to take more than money to turn his life around.

Bob is typical of many people with metabolic syndrome. They're in their current situation because their priorities are upside down, just as Bob's are.

That's one of two common themes I've seen over the years: 1) patients have experienced some symptoms by the time they see me, but they've delayed seeking care; 2) patients have relied on their physician and care team to appropriately meter the level of concern with the findings. And as I mentioned, sometimes that falls short. Your auto mechanic will give you a harder time about how you're caring for your car than your doctor will about how you're caring for your body. I've found that my patients tend to take far better care of their worldly possessions than they take care of themselves. It's frustrating for me to see the neglect that some impose on their own body. When their body breaks down, they're surprised their own neglect has caught up with them. I have not only been caring for patients for over thirty years, but also studying them as well. I am puzzled by why some patients call me at the very first sign of a problem and won't stop asking questions until they get a full explanation, while others simply ignore symptom after symptom and only reluctantly present themselves at the office. Denial is a wonderful defense mechanism against the unpleasant thought that something may be wrong with you. My approach is to make my patients, and all who listen to this message, well-informed consumers of health information, which is a good first start.

Now, it's human nature for people to minimize what they are told. And since the diagnosis usually includes the words "beginnings of" or "a touch of" — "You have the *beginnings* of fatty liver," "You have a touch of diabetes," —a large portion of patients view their situation as less serious than it really is. They're not connecting the dots to understand that "beginning" or "touch of" means the early stage of a disease, and that many of these disorders are progressive, slowly but surely getting worse with time. That progression may take months or years, but it will occur. And, in a sense, they just don't understand how lucky they are. By acknowledging the disease early, there may still be time to change their lifestyle and potentially prolong their life.

The truth is that healthcare seems to take a back seat to practically everything else in life. In fact, a rather absurd analogy that I have been making for the last twenty-five years is that people take better care of their computers than they do of themselves. Microsoft has reported that only 24 percent of computers around the world are still unprotected from viruses.[51] Yet only around 64 percent of adults have an up-to-date tetanus shot, and only 20 percent of adults considered high risk for contracting pneumonia have been vaccinated.[52] The first thing IT help desk personnel ask when someone contacts them about a potential computer virus or malware is whether that person's antivirus program is up to date—and people are regretful to admit that it isn't. Yet 80 percent of the population has not been vaccinated for serious disease, and no one is giving these people a hard time for their lack of vaccination.

Part of the reason for a state of denial is that people don't really understand what their test results mean. They don't understand what it means to have elevated blood sugar, triglycerides, or liver chemistries. They don't understand what it means when an ultrasound reveals a fatty liver, or other irregularities. Again, liver abnormalities often manifest no symptoms even though the lab results reveal them, which can make it even harder to believe there's a problem that needs to be addressed immediately. The liver is not like, for example, the lungs. When people have a chronic cough or are short of breath, they're more likely to think something is wrong with their lungs. They're more likely to go get checked. If someone's hip, or knee, hurts going up a flight of stairs, or their shoulder hurts playing golf, that person is more likely to seek out medicine or a doctor's help. Another common misconception is if there is a lack of pain, or no general loss of function of any particular body part, all is assumed to be fine. In many cases, this approach leads to critical delays in seeking appropriate care, which in turn can result in serious complications and poor outcomes. This is where I feel, by communicating these issues to you, I can make the biggest impact. I call these diseases silent, but deadly. They don't get attention until they manifest symptoms. I don't know whether this is a manifestation of denial or has to do with patients minimizing the importance of these conditions because they don't interfere with their daily life.

So, a part of the solution for dealing with liver disease and metabolic syndrome, and other general health concerns, is to understand how important it is to take care yourself. And that begins by better understanding "normal" body standards and what test results mean.

## Body Mass Index

As I mentioned in chapter one, body mass index (BMI) is a measure of body fat based on a person's height and weight. A high BMI can lead to elevated blood pressure, triglycerides, blood sugar, bad cholesterol levels, inflammation—all precursors to disease. There are a number of good online BMI calculators.

As I mentioned in chapter one, another good way to understand whether your health is within normal standards is to measure your waist-to-hip ratio (the measure of your waist divided by the measure of your hips). The result should not exceed 0.85 for women and 0.9 for men.

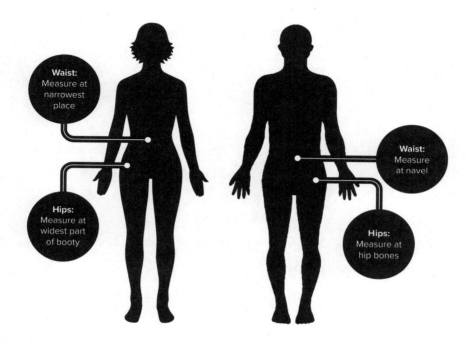

So, if a man is five feet eleven inches and weighs 270 pounds, his BMI is 37.7. That signals obesity, almost morbid obesity. My role, then, is to help him understand his goal should be around 179 pounds, a normal BMI of 25. For the patient, that often seems like an insurmountable hurdle. "I haven't weighed less than 200 pounds since high school," he might say. The truth is that may have been the last time he was metabolically healthy. But that's what it's going to take to be healthy and reduce the risk of metabolic syndrome—or turn it around.

Studies have shown that a lower BMI lowers the risk of chronic disease and death, and that the risk of death increases significantly with weight gain. And it doesn't take much. A BMI of 25 to 27 raises the risk of mortality by 7 percent; 27 to 30 raises the risk by 20 percent; 30 to 35 raises it by 45 percent; and 35 to 40 raises it by 94 percent.[53] Increased weight does matter. The current norms of what people think they should weigh are distorted, and this is impacting how they view themselves and approach the problems they face.

## Cholesterol

As I mentioned previously, there are two kinds of cholesterol: high-density lipoproteins (HDL or "good" cholesterol), and low-density lipoproteins (LDL or "bad" cholesterol). Your risk of cardiovascular disease is greatest when you have *elevated* low-density and *low* high-density cholesterol along with elevated triglycerides. Cholesterol lives in your bloodstream, where it can either protect your body or lead to disease.

Somewhere around one-third of adults, about 71 million Americans, have elevated low-density lipoprotein, or bad cholesterol. Only one in three adults with high LDL cholesterol has the condition under control. As people gain weight and continue to eat poorly, the problem gets worse. The vast majority of people with fatty liver disease die of a cardiovascular event such as a heart attack or stroke.

Total cholesterol levels should be less than 200 mg/dL (milligrams per deciliter). A level of 200–239 mg/dL is borderline high, and 240 mg/dL is high.[54] LDL (bad) cholesterol levels should be less than 100 mg/dL, and HDL (good) cholesterol should be 60 mg/dL or higher.

# Diabetes

Type 2 diabetes affects approximately 9.4 percent of the United States population, with as many as 25 to 40 percent of those with diabetes undiagnosed.[55] Diabetes is a devastating disease, associated with damage to the blood vessels, diabetes accounts for almost 14 percent of US healthcare costs, at least one-half of which are related to complications such as heart attack, stroke, kidney failure, blindness, diabetic foot ulcers, *and fatty liver*.

Accurate testing for diabetes can be performed several ways. Diabetes testing for a diagnosis does not have to involve fasting and has three separate criteria. The first of these criteria concerns fasting glucose, which should be *less* than 100 (the value of 100 is prediabetes, or impaired fasting glucose) The A1c test analyzes the three-month average of the blood glucose level as a percentage, which should be 5.7 percent or less. The oral glucose tolerance test (OGTT) measures the glucose level over a two-hour period. A level of 200 mg/dl or higher confirms a diagnosis of diabetes. Often, when the blood sugar level registers at 105 or 110 mg/dl, the patient believes it's just a "touch elevated and nothing to worry about." As I mentioned in chapter one, there's no such thing as "a touch of diabetes," especially when it's combined with obesity, high cholesterol, or fatty liver. At that point, it's an early warning sign of something more. That's when you need to have a serious discussion with your physician. Repeat the blood sugar test. If it is persistently elevated, you may want to do a hemoglobin A1c test. A hemoglobin A1c, also called glycosylated hemoglobin, is a blood test that will give a roughly sixty- to ninety-day average reading of what your blood sugar has been and may be a better barometer of what kind of a problem you may be dealing with. For people who don't have diabetes, the normal range for the hemoglobin A1c level is between 4 and 5.6 percent. Hemoglobin A1c levels between 5.7 and 6.4 percent mean you have a higher chance of getting of diabetes. Levels of 6.5 percent or higher mean you have diabetes. Based on that test, you may need to go for a glucose tolerance test to further diagnose insulin resistance and/or outright type 2 diabetes. Here again, the take-home message is that slight abnormalities of blood glucose need to be thoroughly investigated. The risk of progression to type 2 diabetes when these labs show glucose levels to be in the prediabetes range is about 5 to 15 percent per year. A slightly abnormal reading does matter and has serious consequences associated with it. Adjusting your diet with reduces calories and serving size is the first step to addressing the blood sugar concerns.

## Liver Tests

Liver tests are sometimes called liver chemistries or liver function tests. The term *liver function tests* is somewhat of a misnomer. These lab values, tied to the liver, do not represent how the liver is functioning. They simply represent a general indication that there is some type of yet-to-be-determined damage or inflammation taking place in the liver. There are several different tests for liver enzymes.

### Alanine Transferase and Aspartate Transaminase

There are numerous reasons why liver chemistries may be elevated. They may be related to a virus, a medication, alcohol, excess iron or copper in the liver, or excess fat. There are also a host of autoimmune diseases that can attack the liver and cause damage to the cells.

Testing for damage or inflammation in the liver looks at the liver enzymes alanine transferase (ALT) and aspartate transaminase (AST). Test results are measured in units per liter (U/L).

There is no correlation between the elevation of the liver chemistries and the severity of damage. For example, based on an upper limit of 40 U/L as normal, a person whose test result is 41 U/L may have just as much damage as someone whose result is 240 U/L, or two hundred points above normal. Any elevation of liver chemistries is a red flag that must be taken seriously and investigated. For most things in nature, a larger number means something greater. That's not the case with liver enzymes. Liver enzymes that are one point above normal are just as serious as liver enzymes that are ten or two hundred points above normal. Getting any level of elevated reading is no time to say, "Well, it's just a couple of points." Elevated liver enzymes need to be carefully evaluated further. Period.

Currently, there is a movement in medicine to lower the upper limit of what's defined as "normal" liver chemistries. That raises a valid concern. If normal becomes the lower twenties range instead of forty, then hundreds of thousands of additional people that now have elevated liver chemistries, under these new guidelines, would need a medical review. According to the National Health and Nutrition Examination Survey (NHANES) database, lowering the norm would result in 36 percent of men and 28 percent of women having elevated liver chemistries as a result of fatty liver and obesity.[56]

At my practice, we consider results within 15 to 20 points of the upper level of normal to be abnormal, depending on other factors. By making this change to "what's normal" for liver chemistries, we have lowered the threshold for concern, and thus further investigation. Despite the fact that patients have been told their liver chemistries are in the upper level of normal and there is no need for concern, we view these levels as abnormal, and uncover serious problems that otherwise would have been ignored.

## Alkaline Phosphatase

Elevated levels of alkaline phosphatase may be an early indicator of a problem with the bile ducts, including certain diseases that destroy the ducts such as primary biliary cholangitis (PBC) or primary sclerosing cholangitis (PSC). Since alkaline phosphatase is also present in bone, disorders of the bones can cause elevation of alkaline phosphatase, completely unrelated to any liver disorder.

## Gamma-Glutamyl Transpeptidase

If elevated alkaline phosphatase is documented in your lab results, then a follow-up test of gamma-glutamyl transpeptidase (GGTP) should be done to determine whether this elevation originated in the liver. GGTP is only located in the liver bile ducts, and very specific. Inflammation of the bile ducts, or any type of obstruction or blockage will raise the GGTP. Sticky bile, or sludge, can elevate the GGTP. Gallstones in the bile ducts and malignant tumors of the bile ducts will also cause an elevation of GGTP. The bile ducts are a network of tubes inside the liver that drain the bile from the liver and gallbladder to the intestines to help with digestion. GGTP is very sensitive and can also become elevated with alcohol use. Based on the results of the alkaline phosphatase and GGTP tests, further investigation may be required through ultrasounds and MRIs.

## Antimitochondrial Antibody

A positive antimitochondrial antibody (AMA) test is diagnostic of PBC. Generally speaking, PBC tends to occur more in young, white females than it does in men. PBC is inflammation of the bile ducts due to an autoimmune disorder, which can lead to more extensive scarring of the bile ducts, blockage of the bile ducts, and ultimately, cirrhosis and scarring of the entire liver, which may necessitate a transplant. Patients who test positive for the AMA have a 95 percent chance of having PBC. PSC, a similar disease of the liver that primarily affects the bile ducts, is very common in people who have inflammatory bowel disease such as Crohn's disease or ulcerative colitis. People with PSC will have a slight elevation of their ALT and AST, along with an elevation of their alkaline phosphatase and GGTP. So, it's possible to have scarring and damage of the bile duct predominantly at first, but not of the liver. There are FDA-approved medicines that can slow the progression of PBC. Like PBC, PSC can eventually lead to cirrhosis and liver failure, necessitating the need for liver transplantation. Unfortunately, an additional concern in those with PSC is the development of cholangiocarcinoma, which is cancer of the bile ducts. Because of the difficulty in detecting this cancer early, many cases are diagnosed in the later stages, when therapy is far less effective. At Houston Methodist Hospital, we have an aggressive protocol for cholangiocarcinoma which involves both chemotherapy and radiation, as well as the added benefit of liver transplantation, when necessary.

## Bilirubin

Elevated bilirubin is what causes jaundice (indicated by yellowing of the skin and eyes), and darkening of the urine. Anything that prevents normal flow of bile through the liver and bile ducts will lead to an elevation of the bilirubin and jaundice. Gallbladder disease, gallstones, hepatitis, and tumors in the liver, bile duct, or pancreas can cause bilirubin elevation. Interestingly, when bile doesn't flow properly through the liver, the stool gets pale and clay-colored. That's because bile, which is usually yellow to green in nature and gives stool its brown color, is missing.

Look at it this way: A mild elevation is an early warning sign and may be the window of opportunity that gives you years to change things around before your condition becomes more serious or irreversible. Don't squander the opportunity. Don't let anyone tell you, "These results might be normal for you." Baloney. That is not the way to look at elevated tests.

## Alpha-Fetoprotein

For liver cancer, also called hepatocellular carcinoma or a hepatoma, the tumor marker is alpha-fetoprotein (AFP). This blood test should be conducted on people that already have chronic liver disease and cirrhosis. The standard guidelines screening for liver cancer are an ultrasound and AFP blood measurement every six months, screening for either the development of a visible abnormality or tumor, and/or a rise in the AFP value. An elevated AFP may be the earliest indicator that cirrhosis has progressed to liver cancer. In most liver conditions, liver cancer is a very late complication, almost exclusively seen after cirrhosis has already set in. Despite the diagnosis of cancer in the liver, based on size and location, liver transplantation may be a curative option. Again, early diagnosis will yield the best outcomes.

## Additional Screening

Once tests identify that your liver enzymes are elevated, it's important to get a differential diagnosis and possible etiologies to determine what exactly is the severity of damage and what is the cause.

Start by considering any additional screening needed. For instance, if you are a baby boomer born between 1945 and 1965, get screened for hepatitis C with a hepatitis C antibody test. If you have a history of blood transfusions before 1992, or if you have a history of intra-nasal or intravenous drug use, tattoos, body piercings, or high-risk sexual contact, then you need to be screened for hepatitis C. Too many people are embarrassed to admit that in college they may have experimented with drugs. Now they're successful pillars of the community, so they don't want their past to come to light by going for a hepatitis C test. So, what do they do? They deny having any risk factors, refuse to get tested, and then lose the opportunity to get ahead of a problem. Treatments for hepatitis C today carry a near 100 percent cure rate.

If you or your parents came from an endemic area for hepatitis B, such as Asia or Africa, you need to be tested. Gay men should be tested, intravenous drug users, people on dialysis, people with HIV, or anyone with a household member who has hepatitis B should also be screened.

Also get screened for hepatitis A, which is spread through the fecal/oral route. Typically, contraction of hepatitis A occurs because of poor hand washing and sanitary practices by food handlers infected with the disease. A negative result is an opportunity to be vaccinated for hepatitis A and B, both of which are safe and very effective.

## Regions where hepatitis B is prevalent:

- ✓ **Pacific Islands**
- ✓ **Africa (excludes Algeria, Egypt, Libya, Morocco, Tunisia)**
- ✓ **Middle East (Jordan, Saudi Arabia)**
- ✓ **Eastern Mediterranean**
- ✓ **Southeast Asia**
- ✓ **Central and Eastern Europe**
- ✓ **Central and South America**
- ✓ **Canada (Northwest Territories, Nunavut, Yukon)**
- ✓ **Denmark**
- ✓ **Greenland**
- ✓ **Alaska**

*The World Health Organization*

If an individual tests positive for elevated liver enzymes and has any other metabolic syndrome characters—obesity, diabetes or insulin resistance, high cholesterol—then an ultrasound may be needed to determine whether or not they have a fatty liver. An ultrasound of the liver is a non-invasive imaging test making use of sound waves, with no risk of radiation, to evaluate the structure of the liver and surrounding organs of the abdomen. Ultrasounds can detect 20 percent or more fat when present in the liver.

Lifestyle should also be considered when liver enzyme levels are elevated. Chronic alcohol use is a very common cause of the liver enzyme elevation. Women should have no more than one drink or alcoholic beverage per day and men should have no more than two.

**I'm often asked what defines a "drink."**

- ✓ **One bottle of beer:** 12 fluid ounces (355 milliliters)
- ✓ **One glass of wine:** 5 fluid ounces (148 milliliters)
- ✓ **One shot of distilled spirits (80 proof):** 1.5 fluid ounces (44 milliliters)

In women, ten to twelve drinks per week, and in men eighteen to twenty drinks per week may cause liver enzyme elevation. What's interesting is that while, for most liver problems, ALT is elevated to a higher degree, when alcohol is the cause, AST levels tend to be greater than ALT by two to one.

## Iron Overload: Hereditary Hemochromatosis

Excess iron in the body can lead to liver disease and cirrhosis, as well as organ damage involving the heart. Hereditary hemochromatosis (HH), in which the body absorbs too much of the iron consumed, remains the most common, identified, genetic iron-overload disorder in Caucasians. Although its geographic distribution is worldwide, it is seen most commonly in populations of northern European origin, particularly Nordic or Celtic ancestry, in which it occurs with a prevalence of approximately one per 220 to 250 individuals. Screening should also look at ferritin levels. Ferritin is a protein that binds to iron in the blood. High levels of ferritin indicate an excess of iron.

Patients whose tests reveal high levels of AST and ALT should also be checked for autoimmune diseases such as rheumatoid arthritis, lupus, or Sjogren's syndrome (which can cause dry mouth and eyes). Connective tissue disorders such as these tend to be more common in women. The concern is that the autoimmune part of the disorder may affect the liver. A test for antinuclear antibody (ANA), and anti-smooth-muscle antibody (ASMA), can determine if an autoimmune disorder is the culprit.

## Rarer Conditions

A number of rarer conditions should be screened for if the liver enzymes tests is elevated. Among these is Wilson's disease, a genetic disorder leading to copper overload in the body. Wilson's disease is more common in young people and older adults and can cause a decrease in IQ and aptitude; youth with Wilson's disease often do poorly in school. Excess copper can be deposited in the brain and nervous system, causing neuropsychiatric problems. Wilson's disease can also affect the liver when too much copper builds up, causing symptoms similar to advanced cirrhosis. The screening test for Wilson's is serum ceruloplasmin, and levels less than 20 mg/dL indicate the presence of the disease. It can also be confirmed with a twenty-four-hour urine copper collection test, which will reveal elevated copper level in the urine, or by an eye exam that looks at the fringe of the eye for copper deposits known as Kayser-Fleischer rings.

Last is a deficiency of alpha-1 antitrypsin (A1AT), which is an inherited disorder that can raise a person's risk of having both liver and lung disease. Abnormally low levels of A1AT protein in the blood may indicate liver and lung disease. Cirrhosis may develop, as well as advanced lung disease, requiring lung transplant.

## Know Your Lab Tests

- ✓ ALT/AST
- ✓ Alkaline Phosphatase
- ✓ GGTP
- ✓ Bilirubin

## Viral Hepatitis

- ✓ Hepatitis A
- ✓ Hepatitis B
- ✓ Hepatitis C

## Hereditary Conditions

- ✓ Hereditary hemochromatosis (iron excess)
- ✓ Wilson's disease (copper excess)
- ✓ Alpha-1 Antitrypsin deficiency

## Bile Duct Disorders

- ✓ Primary Biliary Cholangitis (Anti-mitochondrial antibody)
- ✓ Primary Sclerosing Cholangitis

## Autoimmune Disorders

- ✓ Anti-nuclear antibody (ANA)
- ✓ Anti-smooth muscle antibody (ASMA)

# Medications: Not Always Safe

While some medications are known to cause enzyme elevations, such as the antibiotic Augmentin (amoxicillin/clavulanate) or the antiseizure medicine Dilantin (phenytoin), nearly any medication can cause a liver reaction. One that deserves special attention is acetaminophen. This is the active pain reliever ingredient in Tylenol. For many patients and consumers, certain trade name medicines are grouped together for a specific action they perform. Any time patients are taking a pain reliever for a headache, a sore back, or flu-related fever, they will say, "I'm taking Tylenol" (in a similar fashion, they will also say they are taking Pepcid for their heartburn). In many instances, they are *not* taking Tylenol but, rather, a nonsteroidal anti-inflammatory drug such as ibuprofen. Bottom line: many well-intentioned patients have no idea what they are taking. This is a prescription for serious complications. Regarding acetaminophen, and thus my warning to you, keep in mind the following precautions:

The maximum dose daily is 3,000 mg.

- ✓ Do not take acetaminophen if you consume alcohol, which greatly increases its liver toxicity, possibly causing liver failure and death, with no early warning symptoms.

- ✓ There are over five hundred nonprescription products that contain acetaminophen, increasing the potential for inadvertent overdose.

- ✓ Numerous prescription pain relievers, such as Vicodin, Norco, and Lortab, contain acetaminophen. Taking additional acetaminophen may lead to overdose.

More people are taking natural supplements and being duped into thinking they are safe. These are not investigated or tested by the US Food and Drug Administration (FDA) or any other appropriate body. There is a false sense of security thinking that because a supplement is "natural," it is safe. That is pushed all the time: natural means it's safe, as opposed to a pharmaceutical that is unnatural. What I tell patients is that poison ivy is natural, but you don't want to roll in it. A rattlesnake is natural, but you don't want to ride in a car with one, do you? Just because something is touted as natural does not mean it is good for you. It does not mean it is free of danger. So many of these misperceptions perpetuate themselves, and are widely distributed online. Remember too that many of the pharmaceutical drugs we have today are derived from plants.

## Next Steps

Once the blood work is back, you must be prepared to talk about next steps. That will likely be an ultrasound of the liver and abdomen.

The ultrasound images are created by sound waves. There's no radiation, and no risk to you. The ultrasound gives the size, shape, surface characteristics, and density of the liver. It can determine if the liver is enlarged or has a lumpy surface, which may indicate scarring and the early stages of cirrhosis. Ultrasounds are very sensitive in detecting fat in the liver, and are routinely used for first-line screening. They can see if there are any tumors or cysts in the liver. Ultrasounds can also see whether the appearance of the gallbladder and pancreas are normal and look at the bile ducts to ensure there's no blockage. Doppler studies of the liver and abdomen, done as part of the ultrasound exam, can determine the blood flow into and out of the liver.

In certain conditions, clots, or thrombosis, can develop in the circulation system of the liver.

A more thorough investigation of the liver may include a CT scan, which involves radiation. In most cases, you're going to get the best image of the liver when intravenous contrast (an injected dye) is used. Depending on the situation, MRI with contrast can give an even more high-resolution imaging of the liver, the bile ducts, and the pancreas. Compared to the CT scan, MRI uses a magnet to create the image, and no radiation. Specialized MRI that looks at the bile ducts is magnetic resonance cholangiopancreatography (MRCP). MRCP provides a detailed anatomy of the bile ducts rather than of the liver itself.

Two tests that are relatively new include the NAFLD fibrosis score, a noninvasive scoring system that uses a panel of blood tests to estimate the amount of scarring. The score can help identify patients who might benefit from additional testing such as a liver biopsy or elastography. The latter of these, FibroScan, uses ultrasound technology to calculate the degree of damage and/or fibrosis within the liver. This innovative technology may one day replace the need for a liver biopsy. FibroScan sends a special ultrasound signal into the liver, and that signal bounces back onto the transducer, which is a device held against the skin to give a reading of the stiffness of the liver. A liver that is inflamed and has scar tissue is stiffer, less flexible, and may indicate the potential risk for developing cirrhosis.

A liver biopsy allows for a small piece of the liver to be taken and then analyzed under a microscope with a pathologist. This test may be ordered based on the patient's clinical symptoms and the results of blood tests and imaging. That can give additional information about the underlying cause of the problem and the extent of damage along with a window into what the next one to five years has in store for the patient. There are small risks associated with liver biopsies, but if patients are properly selected, the risk can be further mitigated. In many cases, a biopsy is going to be very important in making the best diagnosis. It will provide information that cannot be gained from the physical exam, laboratory testing, or imaging.

## Listen to Your Body

Again, in the beginning stages of liver disease, there may not be many symptoms. You're just living life and everything seems fine. That's because the liver is different from the heart, lungs, hips, back, or eyes. The liver tends to suffer in silence!

But there are alarming symptoms that cannot be ignored. I mentioned a few in the last chapter; I'm reiterating them here along with others. You must listen to your body and have these symptoms checked out.

- ✓ **Chronic fatigue**. Anytime you have chronic fatigue, get it checked.

- ✓ **Edema (swelling) in your legs and lower extremities**. This could point to a liver problem, especially if the edema is pitting, meaning it's leaving a depression in your skin when you push on the area with your finger.

- ✓ **Unusual rapid weight gain.** This may be a sign of more advanced liver problems.

- ✓ **Increasing abdominal girth.** This is a potentially serious sign of liver disease. (It's also a potential sign of heart disease and congestive heart failure as well.)

✓ **Obvious changes in the skin, eyes, urine, stool**. Recognizable yellowing of the skin or eyes, darkening of urine, or clay-colored stools are potentially ominous signs that you have a problem.

✓ **Blood in the stool**. Countless people, out of a sense of denial, chalk up blood in the stool to hemorrhoids. But if you have a bowel movement and your stool is black, it's certainly a very obvious sign of bleeding, potentially indicating advanced liver disease or other serious disorders of the stomach and intestine.

## The Color of Stool

✓ **Black: Bleeding From The Esophagus or Stomach**

✓ **Maroon: Small Intestine or First Part of Colon**

✓ **Bright Red: Lower Colon and Rectum**

✓ **Anemia.** This is often due to chronic liver disease, kidney disease, or chronic bleeding. Anemia of any kind needs to be investigated thoroughly.

✓ **A low platelet count**. Platelets are the blood cells responsible for clotting. A complete blood count (CBC) test counts white blood cell, hemoglobin (red blood cells), and platelet count. At most labs, a normal count is between 150,000 and 350,000 platelets. Low platelets may lead to more bruising, bleeding gums, or cuts that bleed without stopping. With advancing liver disease and cirrhosis, due to liver scarring and the associated resistance to blood flow *through* the liver, circulating blood in the abdomen is diverted to the spleen where platelets are trapped. The result is a lower than normal platelet count in your bloodstream, and an enlarged spleen.

✓ **Abdominal pain**. People tend to have a pretty high tolerance for abdominal pain, nausea, and vomiting. But abdominal pain that persists for more than a couple of days should be investigated. Pain in the right upper quadrant may be related to the liver or gallbladder. Pain in the lower left quadrant may be related to the colon. Pain on the lower right side may be the appendix. Pain in the middle of the abdomen that radiates to the back may represent inflammation of the pancreas. And pain with eating may represent an ulcer in the stomach or the small intestine.

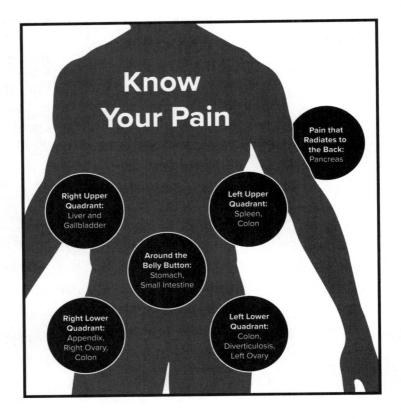

✓ **Persistent constipation or diarrhea**. Again, people are all too accepting of these problems. Constipation or diarrhea that persist needs to be evaluated. Elevated liver chemistries combined with diarrhea may be a sign of undiagnosed colitis and sclerosing cholangitis, which has a very high incidence with inflammatory bowel disease. If you're constipated, it may be due to some other systemic problem that's affecting the liver as well.

✓ **Weight loss**. Unexplained weight loss in general is not necessarily related to a fatty liver problem per se, but weight loss needs to be a red flag of sorts. If you experience unexplained weight loss, there are some warning signs to heed. These include difficulties swallowing, bloating, nausea and/or vomiting after eating, persistent constipation or diarrhea, bright red blood bowel movements, or black and tarry stools.

✓ **Shortness of breath.** When walking up a flight of stairs shortness of breath should not be accepted as normal just because you're getting a little older. There's a fine line here. If you're ninety years old and get a little short of breath when you're going up stairs, that may be more forgivable. But without a host of other health problems, getting short of breath when you walk or climb stairs or exert yourself is not normal.

✓ **Chest pain.** This is not a normal condition to have when you walk or exert yourself. Do not blame it on indigestion or a pulled muscle. If it persists, it needs to be looked at. Call 9-11 immediately.

✓ **Palpitations, skipped heartbeats, a fluttering in your chest.** All of these complaints need to be investigated with your doctor. Don't just go online and try to self-diagnose.

Irregularities of the heart many times may be an indicator of something else wrong in the body. In a worst-case scenario, it may be the only warning you get for a soon to be fatal cardiac event and sudden death.

✓ **Night sweats**. A drenching sweat while you're sleeping may be an indication of an underlying malignancy, infection, or some sort of cancer. Night sweats need to be considered in the context of conditions you're dealing with or medications you are taking. Premenopausal women may have night sweats or sweating episodes. But a fifty-year-old man who has night sweats for no reason needs to get to the doctor.

The bottom line is that your body should be symptom-free. You should not be walking around with pain. And that means being alert to symptoms that you may be having.

Just as people are obsessed with their cars, computers, and gadgets, they need to take a deep interest in their bodies. After all, it's the most important machine anyone has.

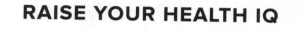

# RAISE YOUR HEALTH IQ

1.  What is the normal body mass index (BMI)?

2.  Your total cholesterol should be below what value?

3.  Alanine transferase and aspartate transferase are blood tests of which organ?

4.  What is the recommended maximum of alcohol beverages a woman can consume each day?

5.  Hemoglobin A1c is a blood test tool to help manage which disease?

# CHAPTER 5

# Take Control Of Your Health—Now

→ *Physician-Patient Communication 101*
→ *The Pill Mentality: Get Over It*
→ *The Greatest Weapon: the Desire to Be Well*

**Twenty-eight-year-old Barb worked** as a teacher's aide. She was single and had no children. At five feet four inches tall and weighing nearly 300 pounds, she was considered morbidly obese. She was also prediabetic and, when tested, was found to have elevated cholesterol and liver enzyme levels. Following those test results, she had an ultrasound that showed she had fatty liver.

When her primary care physician discussed those findings with her, he told her she needed to lose weight or she would probably need a liver transplant within a few years. She was so frightened by that discussion that she did not follow up with him for over a year.

At that point, still not feeling well and dealing with fatigue and depression, she finally went back to the same doctor. She hadn't lost any weight, and a review of updated lab testing revealed no real changes in her health. But while she was interested in learning about her choices for turning her situation around—asking questions about options for weight loss surgery, referral doctors, online information, books, and potential medicines—she found the conversation to be one-sided. In fact, in the middle of the "conversation," the doctor left the room without a word and sent in his medical assistant to complete the visit. The medical assistant was out of the loop on Barb's situation but did what she could to help answer Barb's questions.

Still, Barb was mortified by what had happened and eventually sought me out for further evaluation of her liver and metabolic issues. In her first visit with me, she said we spent more time going over her situation and options than her primary care physician had spent with her over the last few years. This is an all too familiar story I hear repeatedly from patients. As a result of this, I have elected to engage myself, as well as my team, to a course of committing ourselves to listening to what the patients are saying, get a sense for where they stand emotionally, and provide them with the education and compassion they need to be successful in their wellness journey.

The days of a patient going in to see a doctor, spending time talking about health issues, listening as the doctor explains the diagnosis, and then leaving with a fully fleshed-out treatment plan are gone. That's the sad state America's healthcare system is in today.

But that cannot stop patients from pursuing all they need to know to better manage their own health. With all the resources available today, it's time for patients to get involved in better understanding their care. It's time for patients to inform themselves about the treatment they are undergoing, the medications they're being prescribed, and the therapies being used. It's time for patients to be more than passive participants because that's no longer the way to get the best outcomes from care.

In other words, as the patient, you need to be a healthcare consumer. Now, I'm using the phrase *healthcare consumer* even though it is a subject of passionate debate in the media and in the medical field. Those opposed to the use of the word *consumer* point to the fact that, in healthcare, there is little or no room to directly impact the cost or the quality of the product. On some levels, that's true. In the current environment, you may be locked into certain insurance plans. You can't change the doctor's pricing and, in many cases, you can't change the quality of the care you receive.

But I look at the situation from a different perspective. When patients put on their consumer hats, they're putting the healthcare system on notice. As consumers, patients must apply certain consumer basics to the interaction with the doctor, which means demanding better communication, better flow of information, and consequently, better care.

Think of it this way: If you go to a restaurant and order a hot meal that is delivered to your table cold, you're going to demand better service, you're going to demand to get what you paid for. If you don't get it, you won't go back. The same can be true in healthcare. You're paying for the doctor to listen to you and to provide care. That's a service for which you exchange money. If you aren't satisfied with the service, why go back?

As I see it, doctors must be put on notice. They must understand that, unless they and their staff provide better service, better communication, patients are going to go to another facility or another practice. That's why I view patients as consumers of healthcare.

# Physician-Patient Communication 101

The goal, then, is to create a partnership where physicians work to serve patients and educate them about how to take care of themselves, and patients follow through on treatment while working proactively to get themselves healthier—and staying that way. We strive for a win-win proposition. Our patients' problems are related to obesity, metabolic syndrome, and fatty liver, and they aren't eating the way they should. Both medical and lifestyle interventions are required to make things right. Physicians need to be conscious that they are establishing meaningful therapeutic relationships with their patients.

That means a relationship must be built between physician and patient through communication; there must be better communication from the doctor, and more willingness from the patient to do more than just take a pill. Building that relationship means employing some basic measures, which I like to call physician-patient communication 101.

## Set Expectations Early

Especially when seeing a new provider, it's important to go into the first appointment with the mindset of setting expectations for the relationship. First and foremost, there must be an appreciation and respectfulness of the physician and the appointment time, but the patients must also be assertive enough to ensure communication about the type of relationship they expect. That communication must include how much the patients want to be involved with their care, how much they expect to be able to participate in decision making, and how much detail they want about treatment options. For some patients, that means little or no discussion and general instructions from the doctor: "Here's what you have. Here's what I want you to do. Come back and see me in three weeks." For others, that means discussing everything from potential side effects of medication to upfront information about the potential progression of their disease to resources that can be used to gain more knowledge about their condition.

When you set expectations, remember that they must be reasonable. For many patients, that means finding the best fit with a provider within certain parameters. Insurance and household finances may narrow the field of providers. For some patients, the best "fit" is worth the extra out-of-network costs. For others, it means working with a provider who is not the ideal fit for various reasons but meets the patient's healthcare needs satisfactorily.

With less than an ideal fit, it's going to be up to the patients to pursue outside resources to increase their knowledge. Communication will also be key. For instance, if you're the patient and your brother has colon cancer, which has made you especially attuned to the need for regular colonoscopies and results reported in a timely manner and in a way that you can understand, it will be up to you to share those expectations and follow through on communication.

## Get Organized

Building a relationship of effective communication means being organized about care. Prior to the first appointment, patients must be ready to share their health history, including the health of family members. Any prior experience dealing with the disease or condition of concern should also be shared to give the physician a better idea of prior knowledge. For instance, if the patient acted as caregiver for a family member, close friend, or coworker who had the same condition or the patient witnessed the same condition in someone else, that information should be shared. If the diagnosis is, for example, diabetes, and there's a family history of diabetes—both parents had it, mom ended up on dialysis and dad ended up losing his vision—the doctor needs to have that information. It can help the doctor better understand how familiar the patients are with the disease or condition, and how much they might understand about their care on the road ahead. The doctor needs to know whether a diabetic patient already has experience in monitoring blood sugar and handling dietary needs.

With all appointments, patients should be prepared in advance and be organized to make the most of the limited time spent with a provider. That means doing homework about their condition, keeping track and following through on instructions, and informing the doctor about their progress while pursuing recommended treatments. It also means active listening when the doctor is reviewing test results and data. And it means having questions written out ahead of time. For the sake of efficiency, patients should limit those questions to three or four well-pointed questions. The physician just won't have the time to answer fifteen questions.

If multiple physicians are involved, it may be necessary to bring the records from each provider to every appointment, along with an accurate list of medications and current conditions, such as daily blood pressure and blood sugar logs.

In most cases, it's also a good idea—one I highly recommend—for patients to have a family member or friend with them, taking notes. That allows the doctor and patient to communicate undistracted while someone else records the discussion. Patients should ask for clarity on unfamiliar words or conditions and should not be afraid to mention hurdles in the relationship—for instance, when communication is not following the agreed-upon method.

## Know Who to Call

To ensure good communication flow, find out the best way to get answers when needed. Oftentimes answers don't need to come directly from the physician but can be relayed through someone else on the treatment team, such as a registered nurse, nurse practitioner, physician assistant, or medical assistant. Also find out the best form of communication: e-mail, phone calls, voicemail. With today's technology, some practices offer an online resource such as a patient portal where test results and other information can be obtained from a secure website. A number of my patients still send me handwritten letters through the mail that pose questions about their care or their test results. I don't mind these at all. Again, it's all about sharing expectations and setting up the most effective lines of communication.

There are various ways to be connected to a care provider. Take the time to find out what those are and work within them. Don't end up in a healthcare black hole where you are just guessing at answers. Remember that healthcare providers are people too, and they may not understand the relationship early on. For instance, patients who don't feel well during an office visit may be misperceived by the care team as standoffish. If tests show a minor abnormality in a new area, such as a mildly elevated liver chemistry, a care team that only has five minutes per patient, or a doctor who is more concerned about low thyroid and diabetes, may not go into detail about a liver test that is off by one point. In a case like that, it's up to you to follow up in the appropriate manner to get answers. That's why it's important to know how.

## Know When to Move On

Another responsibility you have, as the patient, is to recognize when a physician is not the best fit. The reason to change may be based on style of communication, depth of detail you need about your case, patient-clinic staff interactions, or trust. You shouldn't worry about hurt feelings, a common reason not to change providers. You need to be proactive and receive the care you require and feel most comfortable with.

Most importantly, when it comes to dealing with the multiple characters that make up metabolic syndrome—obesity, diabetes, cardiovascular disease, fatty liver—there are a lot of issues to discuss with a physician in a very short amount of time. As with anything in life, the more moving pieces there are, the more complicated things can become. It's like juggling multiple balls in the air. Diabetes that is out of control is going to make blood pressure more difficult to control. Being overweight will make hypertension harder to control.

**Metabolic syndrome really is a communication stress test for the patient, the doctor, and the care team.**

Elevated cholesterol and triglycerides may require a different medical therapy than the other diseases. Add fatty liver to the mix, and—depending on how much damage has already occurred—the ability to effectively make nutrition changes, implement an exercise program, or control blood sugar may be impaired.

Metabolic syndrome really is a communication stress test for the patient, the doctor, and the care team. But the characters of metabolic syndrome can make it even more important to be able to understand, monitor, and get feedback on all the different systems. And that can create an even greater risk for poor communication and neglect.

## The Pill Mentality: Get Over It

In chapter two, I mentioned how my conversation with patients who have fatty liver and metabolic syndrome includes the need to improve their nutrition and other factors but invariably ends in the request for a prescription to fix their problem.

Basically, they're telling me all the lifestyle changes are just a little too tough to undertake. They're not really willing to start cooking. They're not willing to stop eating fast food for breakfast, lunch, and/or dinner. They would rather just take a pill and make all their problems go away. That's a mentality that must be overcome because, when caught early enough, patients do have the ability to make lifestyle changes to turn around what can be a fatal complication.

Trying to rely solely on medications to turn everything around is a mentality that society has to overcome. Patients who come to the clinic with a shopping bag full of medicines seem unfazed by this. It's not okay to be on fifteen different medicines, especially when at least half of them can be eliminated by making a lifestyle change. Take, for example, heartburn and indigestion. Society has become so accepting of heartburn and indigestion because people know all they must do is take a "purple pill" to relieve their discomfort. They'd rather do that than watch what they eat, keep an eye on their weight, and take a few minutes to exercise. They just want that quick fix from a pill instead of making the effort to change their lifestyle.

In America today, the family physician is under attack in part because a population rife with chronic disease is living longer. Patients are surviving but with cardiovascular disease, congestive heart failure, lung disease, diabetes, kidney disease, endocrine problems, arthritis, and dementia. With so many patients, doctors are squeezed to fill needs. The problem has gotten so bad overseas, in England, the public health service is allowing only one problem to be addressed per visit. So, if you have hypertension, obesity, and a breast lump, then only the most serious of these is addressed. If you want to discuss or be tested for the other problems, you have to come back a week or a month later, with another scheduled appointment.

That is not happening officially here in America. But you have to wonder if, at the subconscious level, a doctor is going to evaluate only the most obvious issue, the problem most apparent, for those patients with multiple troubles. In a single appointment, problems with the least noticeable symptoms are ignored. This is where you need to be proactive in your own health.

That's where metabolic syndrome runs into serious problems. An obese person who goes to the doctor with a migraine is going to get relief for that headache, maybe in the form of a pill. But for the sake of time and resources, the doctor is not going to document the obesity as an active medical problem. That means the patient won't be referred to a dietician or a weight loss and exercise program or a bariatric surgeon.

The reason, I believe, is because the medical profession has become too comfortable with obese patients, not only the morbidly obese but also those with moderate obesity. These patients are the new norm. There are other health issues to worry about when a person is obese: back problems, cholesterol, blood pressure, depression—many that can be resolved with a prescription. But no one is tying everything together and pointing to obesity as the keystone for all the other issues.

Numerous studies have even found that physicians have a negative attitude toward obese patients: they have less respect, provide less information, and express a less positive attitude toward patients who are obese. They view obesity as a self-inflicted problem; obese patients are lazy and don't watch what they eat. As if people should just instinctively know how to eat nutritiously! I've had patients confirm this treatment. They've told me that physicians tend to interrupt patients within fifteen to twenty seconds after the patients begin the conversation. That interruption, they say, means the discussion is over. From that point on, they feel their concerns won't be addressed, so they just nod, take the doctor's orders, and go on their way.

The interesting thing is that the obese patient, the vast majority of the time, has more medical problems, more needs. But the data suggests that physicians are not spending more time with the obese patient who has multiple problems. They're spending the same amount of time with a person who has only one medical issue to address. The obese patient with multiple medical problems is not getting any more face time, which ties back to the economic structure of healthcare today: physicians aren't getting paid any extra for all of the face-time these complex patients require.

But if a patient with persistent high blood pressure that is never addressed in spite of numerous visits to the doctor has a massive heart attack and dies, that could be considered medical malpractice. If the doctor had never in a meaningful way mentioned blood pressure medicine, getting an EKG, checking electrolytes—nothing—that would be viewed as not having met the minimum standard of care. It should be the same for obesity. Obesity is public enemy number one.

It's time to adopt a zero tolerance policy for obesity, fatty liver, or other obesity-related diseases and that goes for patients and providers. We do it for other diseases. When a woman in America has a lump in her breast, the solution is to have it examined and then, if warranted, pursue aggressive treatment. When patients are found to have high blood pressure, they are immediately put on antihypertensives and told to exercise and lower their stress if they are to get it under control. But when it comes to obesity, a medical abnormality, no one is stepping up to say, "Something must be done now." That's why it's up to you, the patient, to no longer endure that kind of *laissez-faire* treatment.

It's time for patients to stand up and say, "Doctor, my BMI is above normal and I don't know how to get it down. I need help. I need a referral to a nutritionist or a dietician. I need to know the best online and local resources." The patient-physician relationship needs to be a partnership to address and overcome obesity with nutrition, exercise, and lifestyle changes before it becomes one of the characters of metabolic syndrome. Somebody has to connect those dots. Then the discussion about what to do can start.

## The Greatest Weapon: The Desire to Be Well

Besides hope, the greatest weapon that we have as humans is the desire to get well, the desire to feel better. That desire can keep people from becoming so frustrated and disillusioned that they give up trying to find a solution to their healthcare issues.

There's no doubt there are conditions that are life ending. There are certain malignancies that despite the best attitudes, eating right, exercising, following medications and therapies, and good communication, will cut a person's life short. But for people with a chronic medical condition, it's important to stay engaged as a healthcare consumer. It's important to be armed with the information to make better decisions. And it's important to have a very healthy, therapeutic relationship with a physician and care team. Having everyone aligned, a healthy environment, and a positive mental attitude will maximize the chances of a much better outcome.

As a healthcare consumer, you must adopt a zero-tolerance policy. You've got to step up and be proactive about your care. Learn to "take it like a man (or woman)" when it comes to hearing what you need to do to turn your health around. All too often I hear that patients are insulted when a physician labels them as obese. Follow recommendations or find another provider whose treatment you feel better suits your needs. Ask questions in the time allotted during a visit and follow up in the best manner possible.

Taking an active role in your health means learning how to eat better and that starts with the point of sale. In the next chapter, I'm going to share insights to help you begin to better understand the food choices you make.

## More Continuing Medical Education on Obesity-Related Disorders

As a healthcare provider, I sometimes wonder if what doctors need is more continuing medical education

(CME) on obesity-related disorders. The current requirements for CME vary from state to state, and some state medical boards do not require any ongoing CME. In Alabama, for example, twenty-five hours of CME are required per year, while California requires 150 hours within a three-year period, and Kentucky requires sixty hours every three years.

I feel there's a need to develop a curriculum that is universal across all states can bring everybody up to speed on metabolic syndrome, liver disease, and all the complicating factors, and establish universal resources for patients. Since obesity is public enemy number one, maybe the solution is to have dedicated courses in obesity and nutrition. In the state of Texas, physicians are required to have one hour of ethics. I'm not saying ethics is not important, but more people are going to die directly from obesity than from doctors who have ethical problems.

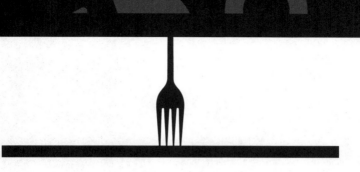

## RAISE YOUR HEALTH IQ

1. What's the maximum number of prepared questions
   you should have when you visit your physician?

2. What benefit is there to having a family
   member or friend accompany you to the
   appointment with your doctor?

3. What is the pill mentality?

4. What negative attitudes do physicians
   have to obese patients?

5. Why is the family physician under so much stress?

# CHAPTER 6

# Food Games: Man Food Vs. Earth Food

→ **Start with a Plan**
→ **Food Industry Tactics**
→ **Understanding Label Claims**
→ **A Serving Size Is How Much?**
→ **Man Food, Earth Food**
→ **Right the Ship**

**"Dr. Galati, we've** really made a conscious decision to eat better this year." It's nice to hear my dear patients say this to me, and I get the satisfaction that a conversation we had earlier in the year, or a recommendation I offered them, made an impression on them. They have realized that a large part of their health issues stems from poor food choices, overeating, lack of exercise, and a general lack of commitment to taking their health into their own hands. Unfortunately, there is a *but* to this story. These patients are *really trying* to eat better and make better decisions, *but* what they are selecting at the market is of no value to them, and in some cases, their proactive approach to better health is actually making them a little worse off than before.

With these patients, as with so many others, terrible mistakes are being made because of the difference between what's perceived as good or healthy food, and what's perceived as bad or unhealthy. Here are some actual patient statements demonstrating what I mean:

**Patient perception.** "Bob and I have eliminated all Dr. Peppers, and instead, we drink organic apple juice throughout the day." The perception? Dr. Pepper: "bad." Organic juice: "good."

**Reality check.** The four servings of juice per day they each reported consuming equals close to 500 calories, 120 grams of carbohydrates, and 96 grams of sugar. By comparison, three Snickers candy bars have a total of 735 calories, 79 grams of carbohydrates, and 65 grams of sugar. Too often, juice is perceived as being healthy because it's usually derived from some sort of fruit or vegetable. But additives for flavor and preservation methods tend to make juices one of the less healthy choices a person can make. Fiber and other nutrients are usually removed from juice, compared to the fruit in its natural state.

**Patient perception.** "We have also started to eat more salad with dinner. Besides the greens and onions, our new favorite dressing is Newman's Own Creamy Caesar."

**Reality check.** Salad is a good addition to a healthful diet, right? Unfortunately, all the extras that people toss in or spoon on add up the calories and bad-for-you mistakes. In this case, the serving size for the dressing is a mere two tablespoons. But how many people stick to that minimal serving? Most drown their salad with three times that amount, supplying them with 510 calories, 54 grams of fat, and 1,020 milligrams of sodium.

**Patient perception.** These patients reported that their vegetable consumption was also on the rise. "Mashed cauliflower—like you suggested—as a substitute for mashed potatoes. We like the frozen Green Giant variety." When asked how much they eat, I was told, "Bob and I split the box."

**Reality check.** There are four-and-a-half servings per box. This vegetable upgrade alone equaled 180 calories, 855 milligrams of sodium, and 12 grams of fat.

Too often, well-intentioned consumers (and patients of mine) are confused as to what to select when they get to the market, and have a false sense of doing the right thing with regard to nutrition and management of obesity and metabolic syndrome. Organic fruit juice is not a healthy substitute when you are removing soda from your diet; while most salads are healthful, the dressing quickly makes it a nutritional disaster; and although some frozen vegetables are acceptable, processing adds far too much salt, and the serving size is deceitful. Who knew? These are the games food manufactures play, and you need to know the rules before you start playing.

People generally have an idea of what foods are good and bad for them. But for those who are less accustomed to making better choices, getting into a better position is where they fall short. For instance, it's easy to believe that since fruit is, generally, good for you, it should also be good when turned into juice. After all, it's natural, low in fat, and has some sort of healthy benefit. People are easily sucker-punched into buying it. "Wow, look at me," they say, "I'm really doing good." But on closer analysis, the actual product and the amount of it that's consumed reveal that it's often a worse choice.

Turning around metabolic syndrome relies on your being a better-informed consumer when shopping for the foods you and your family consume. That's the only way we're going to get a handle on obesity, type 2 diabetes, and fatty liver in children. We need to address the horrifying truth that today's children are not going to live as long as their parents, and that, as forty-five- to fifty-year-old adults, they are going to have lives rife with chronic illness. Yes, there's a role for medical and surgical intervention. Yes, we need the great American healthcare system. But it's going to take intervention and prevention, not just pills and therapies and surgery, to turn back the metabolic syndrome tide that's headed our way.

## Start with a Plan

Being a better consumer involves a fair amount of preplanning before stepping inside a supermarket. Without that planning, it's easy to be caught up in the gravitational pull of a supermarket, to be swayed by what's being pitched to you.

As I mentioned in chapter two, supermarkets are set up to influence what people buy, how much they spend, how much time they hang out there. It's all very carefully orchestrated by the supermarket, playing a little bit on the psyche. Food industry marketers realize people are busy, have little time, and need to get in, get something to eat, and get out. To entice shoppers to buy, they have a number of tricks up their corporate sleeves. They appeal to customers' senses from the moment they enter. Once inside, the bright lights, bright colors, and pleasing music, all make for an experience that invites customers to linger longer.[57]

In chapter two, I discussed the rise in convenience food. With all today's pressures on the two-income family, and everyone too busy to cook and too busy to clean up, supermarkets have responded with an increasing number of premade, ready-to-go foods that require minimal or no prep work.

I also mentioned briefly that these foods have an additional expense: it costs more when you let someone else do the prep and clean up. You're paying for convenience, but the price you're also paying is more salt, more calories, and possibly, more fat. Keeping weight in check and reversing chronic disease relies on taking control of the food being consumed. That's a role that capable individuals should never turn over to anyone else.

There are ways to resist the supermarket gravitational pull. Here are a few tips:

**Have a plan.** Before leaving home, lay out a three-, five-, or seven-day menu that addresses, for the whole family, breakfast, lunch, dinner and/or snacks that you'll have throughout the week.

**Make a detailed shopping list.** Nothing will give you better results and a winning strategy than going to the store with a well-thought-out shopping list that includes all the ingredients you need for the week's meals along with the snacks and/or added condiments, spices, herbs, milk, eggs, and so on. Check the list to ensure it is complete. Look over your week's menu, and check the fridge, freezer, and pantry to ensure you have all the items you need for the recipes you're planning to prepare. Do you need more balsamic vinegar? Do you need more fresh tomatoes? Do you need an avocado? If so, add those to the list.

**Never go to the supermarket hungry.** Before shopping, have a light meal or nutritious snack, and/or eight to sixteen ounces of water. The goal is to satisfy your appetite *before* you get there so your senses don't tell you to buy cupcakes as soon as you walk in the door.

**Make yourself a deal.** Make a deal with yourself that you are not going to buy anything that is not on your list—and stick to it. Supermarkets are banking on impulsive buying. They set up the bakery so that, as soon as you walk in, the scent of baked goods hits your sense of smell, drawing you over in hopes that the visual appeal of the cakes, cookies, and donuts will entice you to buy. You have to realize that and not fall into the trap.

**Avoid end caps.** End caps are the displays on the ends of the aisles that often jut out a little. Items are strategically placed on end caps with the impulsive buyer in mind. Those items may be chips or soda or another type of junk food, but not cauliflower or broccoli or something healthy. Typically, they are cheap but high-profit-margin products. The idea is that as you're walking along in the store, you'll see something on an end cap that entices you to reach out, grab it, and toss it into your basket.

**Set a time limit.** Since supermarkets are designed to keep you shopping and buying items that are not on your list, as part of your planning, give yourself a time constraint.

For instance, if you're shopping once a week, look at your list and determine how long you think it will take to pick up those items—forty-five minutes, thirty minutes, whatever you can accomplish in a minimal amount of time. The longer you linger, the more likely you're going to buy items you really do not need.

**Skip the free samples.** Avoid taste-testing the free food samples being given out at the store. It's easy to think of those as a light snack, but once you get a taste of that highly seasoned, hyperflavored food, there is a pretty good chance that you'll head over to the frozen food section and pick up the product. Remember that if it's not on the menu for the week, it's not on your shopping list, so don't be duped into buying junk you don't need.

**Minimize the number of trips.** With planning, you'll be able to minimize the number of trips you need to make to the store, reducing the chances of getting sucked in and picking up unneeded items. Shopping only once a week forces you to be more organized.

Compared to a convenience store or food mart at the gas station, the grocery store may have a better reputation for fresh vegetables, fruit, dairy, and meat. But don't be entirely fooled by that. The vast majority of calorie-dense, low-nutrient foods are sold in supermarkets. If you go in better informed, realizing the pitfalls, you will not step on the landmines that are planted throughout the entire store. Remember that you must know the rules of the game.

# Food Industry Tactics

Food industry marketers have a number of tactics to perpetuate the cycle of buying food that is unhealthy for you. For instance, super- market managers know people want and like fast food. To capture these dollars, they have added fast-food products to their frozen sections, hoping people will buy these products instead of driving to the restaurant counterpart. These products are geared to the low-prep meal generation.

For instance, in the frozen-food section of the supermarket you'll find Arby's seasoned curly fries, Whataburger potato sticks, Boston Market sweet-and-sour chicken, Nathan's hot dogs, Friday's potato skins—all sorts of fast-food products you can pick up while you're shopping and take home and microwave in the confines of your home.

I've made no bones about how I feel about fast-food restaurants (see chapter two). They are popular in large part because of their drive- through windows. It's easy to grab a meal with no cooking and no cleanup involved. People don't even have to leave their cars.

Now that grocery chains have figured out that people will pay for convenience, they're stepping up to the plate and are even becoming a tremendous threat to fast-food restaurants. Their ready-to-go, cooked-to-order, and hot buffets are designed to cater to the on-the- run consumer. There is a certain perception that maybe, just maybe, since a grocery store sells vegetables, its fast-food choices might be healthier alternatives. But that isn't always true. For starters, portions tend to be more than a single serving, and the self-serve buffets let you load up with choices that are more pleasing to the eye than they are nutritious. The food, in general, is usually saltier, more carb laden, and more calorie dense.

Those grocerants I mentioned in chapter two are designed to blur the lines between shopping and eating, acting as destinations more than just supermarkets. They want you to hang out in the supermarket so you'll buy more—and ultimately, eat more. There's no marketing of any sort to curb what you're eating and how much. In short, they are fostering bad health behaviors that are promoting obesity, metabolic syndrome, and fatty liver.

No matter how you slice and dice it, it's still better—and cheaper—to eat at home.

One final word about grocery stores. They are in business to be profitable and follow the rules of a free enterprise market. They employ millions of Americans and are part of our local communities. My message is simply to be aware that what you buy and consume will influence your health and wellness. Grocery stores sell all you need to eat the picture-perfect diet, one that combats obesity and metabolic syndrome. If you remain uninformed, you can buy products that will make you sick and do nothing for your long-term, disease free state. You have to be your own advocate when it comes to your health.

## Understanding Label Claims

Three categories of claims are currently used on food and dietary supplement labels in the United States: 1) health claims, 2) nutrient content claims, and 3) structure/function claims. Health claims describe a relationship between a food, food component, or dietary supplement ingredient and reducing the risk of a disease or health-related condition. Nutrient content claims are used to describe the percentage of a nutrient in a product relative to the daily value. Structure/function claims were authorized under the Dietary Supplement Health and Education Act and describe the effect of a dietary supplement on the structure or function of the body.

It is my strong opinion that most claims on labels are primarily developed as a marketing ploy, and not necessarily developed for the betterment of the community at large. The manufacturers are anticipating that the consumer is impressed with the claim, and in the spirit of health and wellness, selects their product because of the perceived benefit. These food manufacturers are investing millions of dollars to have these claims printed on the food labels because of the marketing advantage, improved public perception of these products, and ultimately, increased sales and revenue.

Please note: The vast majority of products labeled with such claims are processed foods, which come prepackaged in a container of some sort (box, can, carton, bag, bottle, etc.). No one is pushing the health benefits of carrots.

Let me break down the three types of claim.

## Health Claims

Health claims are based on a very high standard of scientific evidence and significant scientific agreement. There are very few food products and supplements with health claims, because most foods and supplements simply do not meet the established standards or have never been scientifically researched. However, health claims related to various foods involve a complex and highly regulated government process that, by its very nature, is not consumer and patient friendly.

According to FDA guidelines,

*Health claim means any claim made on the label or in labeling of a food, including a dietary supplement, that expressly or by implication, including "third party" references, written statements (e.g., a brand name including a term such as "heart"), symbols (e.g., a heart symbol), or vignettes, characterizes the relationship of any substance to a disease or health-related condition. Implied health claims include those statements, symbols, vignettes, or other forms of communication that suggest, within the context in which they are presented, that a relationship exists between the presence or level of a substance in the food and a disease or health-related condition.*[58]

How can you, the consumer, even begin to understand such legal mumbo-jumbo? Putting it simply, a processed food manufacturer cannot in any way shape or form make *any* claims that the product prevents or treats disease without the approval of the FDA.

Health claims are required to be reviewed and evaluated by the FDA prior to use. An example of an authorized health claim is: "Three grams of soluble fiber from oatmeal daily in a diet low in saturated fat and cholesterol may reduce the risk of heart disease. This cereal has 2 grams per serving." The process for developing these health claims is mired in hundreds of thousands of pages generated by the FDA. There is the tendency, as a result, for patients and consumers to be confused about the meaning of these claims, leading to improper selection of a food, based on a series of false assumptions.

Some labels use health claims to align certain foods with a healthy diet and well-balanced diet, stating in a roundabout way that they may help lower the risk of certain diseases such as cancer, heart disease, stroke, and osteoporosis. Examples of this type of health claim include the following:

- ✓ A healthy diet rich in vegetables and fruit may help reduce the risk of some types of cancer.

- ✓ A healthy diet low in saturated fats and transfats may reduce the risk of heart disease.

- ✓ A healthy diet containing foods low in sodium and high in potassium may reduce the risk of high blood pressure, a risk factor for stroke and heart disease.

- ✓ A healthy diet with adequate calcium and vitamin D and regular physical activity helps to achieve strong bones and may reduce the risk of osteoporosis.

- ✓ Plant sterols help lower cholesterol.

## Nutrient Content Claim

A nutrient content claim is an FDA-approved word or phrase on a food package related to the nutritional value of the food, such as "low calorie" or "fat-free." Examples of nutrient content claims include:

- ✓ low calorie: 40 calories or less per serving
- ✓ reduced-calorie: at least 25 percent fewer calories per serving than the original food
- ✓ light or lite: one-third fewer calories or 50 percent less fat per serving (If more than half the calories are from fat, the fat content must be reduced by 50 percent.)
- ✓ sugar-free: less than one-half gram sugar per serving
- ✓ reduced-sugar: at least 25 percent less sugar per serving than the original food
- ✓ fat-free: less than one-half gram of fat per serving
- ✓ low-fat: three grams of fat or less per serving

- ✓ decaffeinated
- ✓ reduced-fat: at least 25 percent less fat than the original food
- ✓ gluten-free

## Structure/Function Claim

Labels of functional foods (foods that contain extra doses of nutrition) and other products claiming to be dietary supplements are largely unregulated. This allows them to make misleading, unsubstantiated (but legal) claims.

A health or nutrient claim and a claim on functional food may look similar, but you must learn the difference. A health claim is well researched, reliable, and approved by the FDA (e.g., "may reduce the risk of heart disease").

Although deceptively similar, a structure/function claim is not supported by scientific evidence, is far less regulated, and must be worded so that is does not mention a specific disease (e.g., "promotes a healthy heart," "builds strong bones," improves memory," "slows aging," or "provides a variety of health benefits").

The following type of FDA disclaimer must be included on the label: "This statement has not been evaluated by the Food and Drug Administration. This product is not intended to diagnose, treat, mitigate, cure or prevent any disease."

To further complicate the matter, wording by the FDA admits that you, the consumer, must weigh the claim and make a decision. An example from FDA documents,

*It may not be possible always to draw a bright line between structure/ function and disease claims. You should look at the objective evidence in your labeling to assess whether a claim explicitly or implicitly is a disease claim. For example, a statement may not mention a disease but may refer to identifiable characteristic signs or symptoms of a disease such that the intended use of the product to treat or prevent the disease may be inferred. It is important that you keep in mind two things. First, the context of the statement, decided from information on the label and in other labeling will determine if the statement is considered to be a disease claim. Second, foods may not bear disease claims, explicit or implied, unless the claim has undergone premarket review by FDA and has been authorized or approved under the rules for health claims or drugs, as appropriate.[59]*

Such complicated statements further add to the overwhelming confusion, and general deceptive practices that negatively impact the consumer. Make no mistake. These efforts for health claim labeling have nothing to do with making Americans healthier. To the contrary, they are adding to their poor health and disease states.

## A Serving Size Is *How Much*?

In addition to all the health claims on labels, consumers are often confused about serving size. That applies to everything from dairy creamers to snack foods to portions on a plate. Again, I'm talking about processed foods. For the most part, fresh or freshly cooked vegetables and fresh fruits are exempt from my discussion. While some fruits are higher in calories—dried fruits or, as I mentioned, fruit juices, for instance—I'm not too worried about someone getting obese eating too many fresh vegetables.

The key is to understand that avoiding obesity means living within certain guidelines. You cannot just eat whatever you want until you are full and expect to maintain a healthy weight. You must equip yourself with the knowledge of how much you can eat based on calories and other ingredients in food. And that's knowledge that changes over time. For instance, in 1980, a turkey sandwich had about 320 calories. Today, there are around 820 in a typical turkey sandwich. A soda back then was 85 calories, now it's 250.[60]

Using your hand as a measure of serving size:

- ✔ One thumb is a serving of peanut butter (1 tablespoon)
- ✔ One flat palm is a single serving of whole-wheat bread (1 slice)
- ✔ One cupped handful is a single serving of noodles (1/2 cup)
- ✔ One fist is a single serving of dry cereal (1 cup)[61]

The truth is it can be difficult to stay within the guidelines when it comes to serving sizes. How many nights have you finished off an entire pint of ice cream in one sitting? A single serving of Cool Ranch Doritos is only about twelve chips. Twelve chips and you're looking at 150 calories, 70 fat calories, 18 grams of carbs, and 180 mg of sodium. Based on a diet of 2,000 calories a day, it may be worth considering something more filling and with fewer calories. The same number of raw baby carrots equals only 30 calories, no fat, 7 grams of carbs, and 66 mg of sodium. And for desert, there's one serving of Oreo cookies that's 160 calories, five grams of saturated fat, 25 grams of carbs, and 70 mg of sodium. Or, there's a whole apple at 95 calories, 0 grams of saturated fat, 25 grams of carbs, and 2 mg of sodium.

The key is to read the nutrition label. Unfortunately, according to the US Food and Drug Administration, serving sizes have changed over time to more closely reflect how much people actually eat and drink. While a pint of ice cream used to be four servings at 200 calories each, today there are three servings in a pint at 270 calories each. And while soda used to come in a twelve-ounce bottle (one serving, 120 calories), today one serving is a twenty-ounce bottle at 200 calories.[62]

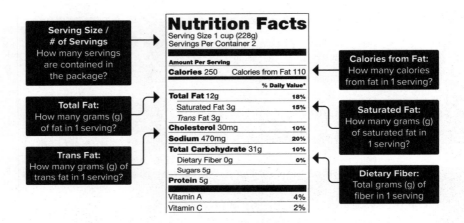

Understanding food labels is a key part of wellness and health.

Remember that 3,600 calories equal one pound of body weight. If you're not exercising or working off many calories in a day, and you're consuming more than the standard diet of 2,000 calories a day, you're going to put on the pounds. Think about that the next time you pick up a bag of chips for lunch. Can you only eat a half a bag in one sitting?

Now, an occasional extra 100 calories here and there is not going to make the difference between being normal weight and healthy and being obese and diabetic. But if you eat an extra 300-calorie serving of chips and cookies every day for lunch, it can. Over the course of a week, 300 extra calories a day is 2,100 calories. So, staying within the label guidelines is key to tracking what you're doing when it comes to servings. Remember that an excess of approximately 3,500 calories will result in a pound of weight gain.

Again, as I mentioned in chapter two, don't be fooled by erroneous labeling designed to make you think something is healthier for you than it is. I hear all the time from patients who are struggling to understand the difference between good and bad foods. When it comes to misleading labels, some of my favorites are:

- ✓ **Pop Tarts.** It would seem like a no-brainer that Pop Tarts are a poor choice in breakfast foods. But parents are often fooled by claims that these sugary breakfast foods are "a good source of vitamins and minerals." What exactly does this mean? The vitamins and minerals are added back by using enriched flour, supplying B1 (thiamine), B2 (Riboflavin), folic acid, B6 (Pyridoxine), Vitamin A, and iron. Supplying a measly 10 percent of these vitamins is laughable.

- ✓ **Eggos.** Parents appreciate the ease that Eggos toaster waffles bring to the breakfast table. But regardless of the claim that they are an "excellent source of calcium," they are also loaded with sodium: 360 mg for two waffles.

- ✓ **Banquet pot pies.** Sodium is a pitfall of most frozen dinners as well. A single Banquet pot pie has 1,000 mg of sodium—bad news for someone with hypertension on a low-sodium diet of 1,500 mg per day.

- ✓ **Blue Bell Ice Cream.** Delicious? Yes, absolutely. Good for you? Not so much. One serving (a half cup—who can eat only a half cup?) is 200 calories, with half of those calories in fat, including 7 grams of saturated fat and 35 mg of cholesterol.

The key is to get educated, enlightened, and most importantly, realize the pitfalls and the trickery designed to make a product look more appealing, to make a product seem healthier than it really is. So you, the consumer, must be aware of what you're doing when it comes to the food you eat. You must be vigilant when shopping, reading labels, and considering serving sizes.

Above all, you must be honest with yourself and with your doctor. If you come to me, weighing 290 pounds, with prediabetes and high blood pressure, I'm going to know you're not eating only a salad every day for lunch. You may be having a cup or two of lettuce, but if you're slathering on the dressing and garnishing with raisins, croutons, bacon bits, and other goodies, you're defeating any attempt you're making at trying to eat healthy. You did not get to be 295 pounds eating romaine lettuce for lunch and dinner every night. No way. You're eating lousy food.

**In my own way, I'm trying to turn around metabolic syndrome one family at a time. If you want to get healthy, if you want to raise your Health IQ, go to DRJOEGALATI.COM**

If my nurse practitioner and I were to drop in unannounced tonight, what would we find in your refrigerator, your freezer, your cabinets? When I'm talking to patients, and their spouse is present, usually one will blame the other for buying the less than nutritious foods in the house—but I know better. So, I often ask patients to take photos of the contents of their cabinets, fridge, and freezer, and I'll conduct a spot analysis for them. Two cases of Dr. Pepper? You've got to get rid of that stuff—now.

# Man Food, Earth Food

There are a lot of excuses for not eating healthy: the cost of fresh food, the time involved in preparing it, the cleanup, and on and on and on … but there are so many benefits to eating healthy food that it perplexes me why people don't. Why doesn't a light bulb go off for those people who are facing potentially deadly illnesses—heart, liver, kidney, cardiovascular, neurologic—to say, "It's time to do something now. I will do anything to make me better."

When it comes to eating healthier food, one way to begin is simply by understanding the difference between man-made food, which I refer to as man food and earth food. Man-made food is anything that is processed. It's food that comes in a container (box, can, carton, etc.). It's food that started out healthier, but has had so many ingredients added to it that you would swear it was a chemistry project. In the process, all the healthy stuff has been stripped out of it—nutrients and fiber and other elements that keep you healthy. Remember that food manufacturers want you to do minimal work to chew and swallow their products and the best way they can do that is to strip out of it the fiber and all the properties that made the original food healthy.

Instead, opt for earth food, which is food that comes from the ground and food that had a mother (thanks to Chuck Garcia for this terminology). As Michael Pollan said in his great book *Food Rules: An Eater's Manual,* "Eat only foods that will eventually rot." If it was made in a factory where people wear white coats and masks, then it's likely been chemically altered. Food with a shelf life of months to years needs to be eliminated from your household.

# Right the Ship

It's time to right the ship. That starts with the meal prep, menu planning, a food list, and a strategy for going to the supermarket and avoiding the landmines. That's followed by understanding calories, unrealistic or deceptive health claims, and serving sizes. And it's about eating only earth food and staying away from man food.

One way to eat better is to grow your own food. Start off in a simple way by planting an herb garden. Some herbs can be grown indoors, while some areas of the country allow for them to survive outdoors year-round. Rosemary, basil, parsley, chives—these can inspire you to incorporate herbs and their flavors into the foods you're making.

Once you see how easy it is to grow herbs, try starting a small garden outdoors. Even a tomato or pepper plant in a container garden can be fun. From there, consider starting a community garden, which can be a great way to work with neighbors and watch your veggies—and your friendships—grow.

Fresh veggies and fruits can also be purchased through local farmers or at a farmer's market. Foods purchased straight off the farm are fresher, more flavorful, and can come in some unique varieties. Buying local lets you know where your food comes from, instead of purchasing something that was green when it was flown from thousands of miles away and ripened on the store shelf.

Ideally, I hope to see the day when grocers, because of their position in the community, work on educating the community to not just buy more of their products but establish a well-rounded, noncommercial approach to nutrition and wellness. That's where we need to go.

Whatever you decide to do, commit to living more healthily. You have nothing bad to lose and a good life to gain.

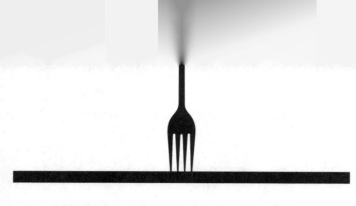

## RAISE YOUR HEALTH IQ

1.  What is the difference between
    man food and earth food?

2.  How many calories are contained in
    four servings of fruit juice?

3.  What are supermarket end caps?

4.  Why should you minimize the number of
    trips to the supermarket each week?

5.  What are grocerants?

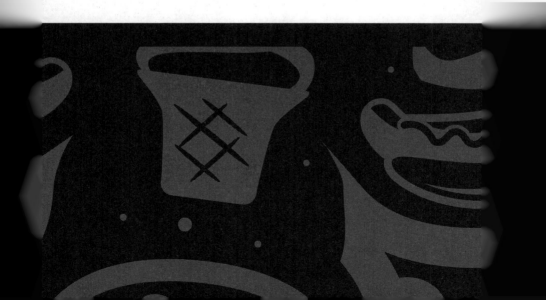

# CHAPTER 7

# The Kitchen— And Family— Revival

➔ *A Healthy Environment*
➔ *It's a National Problem*
➔ *Evolving the Picky Palate*
➔ *Meal Planning: The Best Strategy for Healthier Eating*
➔ *Bring Back the Dinner Party*
➔ *The Great American Produce Giveaway*
➔ *It's Time to Get Over the Fear*

**In the Murphy** household, Karen had largely taken care of the family meals. For years, she did the meal planning, grocery shopping, and meal preparation on her own. By any account, she was comfortable in the kitchen and enjoyed food preparation. Over time, she had learned ways to feed the family healthier food, so the menus had evolved from the standard American diet (SAD) to foods that were organic, fresh, and made from scratch. Karen was aware of the value of her home cooking efforts, and the long-term benefits of this cooking method for her husband and their three boys.

Then Karen's husband, Jim, who always appreciated the food she prepared, was introduced to the Big Green Egg (BGE), a ceramic grill that burns lump coal and can cook a wide range of foods at various temperatures. Always a fan of the conventional backyard grilling experience, this new cooking sophistication took him to a new level. Before long, Jim was taking over a large chunk of the family meal planning. Every day, he looked for new foods to prepare on his grill, even smoking some of Karen's vegetables for the entire family to enjoy. He scoured the Internet daily for new ways to cook anything in his BGE, talking with other BGE colleagues and enthusiasts, collecting cooking tips. Soon, his passion for cooking was contagious. After a while, he mastered this new grilling technique, and the family began to invite others over for meals that featured Jim's latest creations. Soon the couple's three boys were joining in the enjoyment by helping to prepare meals, sharing ideas for menus, and even learning to shop for healthy selections at the grocery store.

---

## Defining Organic Fruits and Vegetables

**Organic crops must be grown without the use of synthetic pesticides, bioengineered genes (GMOs), petroleum-based fertilizers, and sewage sludge-based fertilizers. Organic livestock raised for meat, eggs, and dairy products must have access to the outdoors and be given organic feed. They may not be given antibiotics, growth hormones, or any animal by-products.**

---

Not only did Jim's participation make for a more family-oriented activity, taking some of the responsibility off Karen's plate, but it also gave the family a chance to come together over the food planning and preparation, and, ultimately, to bring others together for social interaction over an enjoyable meal. Cooking at the Murphy house went from being Karen's daily responsibility to being an enjoyable activity for the entire family.

That sharing of the responsibility by all members of the family is the winning strategy that I see in patients—and people who are not my patients—who understand the value of good food and who get excited at the prospect of healthier meals.

For some families, cooking almost becomes a team sport. As with any team sport, everyone has a designated role, and knows how each team member interacts with the others. While one member of the team does the shopping, others provide input on the meal planning, and another oversees the cooking, deciding who cuts the veggies, who grills the meat, who mans the stove, who sets the table. It's more difficult to sustain the effort to cook nutritiously at home if one family member is saddled with 100 percent of the planning, shopping, and preparation of the meals. The key is to get everyone involved in a coordinated play. Just as a football game isn't won by the quarterback alone, a family meal works best when everyone contributes.

## A Healthy Environment

I mentioned earlier how parents are concerned about their kids when it comes to bullying, bicycle safety, seat belts, talking to strangers, and ensuring they get fair treatment at school, but when it comes to nutrition, they don't bat an eye when their children want to eat low-nutrition, low-fiber, unhealthy foods. Yet there is overwhelming evidence that children mimic their parents, including in regard to nutrition. Parents who eat poorly, never cook, and don't know the difference between a zucchini and an eggplant may pass on that same knowledge, or lack thereof, to their kids. That can lead those children down the road to obesity and other diseases that start off in early childhood and end up as metabolic syndrome in adults. When kids are in an unhealthy environment, without the proper guidance, they don't know any better. They're bombarded by friends who eat poorly, by TV commercials that tout unhealthy foods, and by an Internet with less-than-ideal standards.

Better eating and better health begin with mom and dad. It's up to parents to make better food choices and a better environment for healthy living instead of just grabbing a fast-food burger after soccer practice. And it's up to parents to teach their children the merits of good health and eating well. It's time to get back to creating a family environment of healthy habits that kids want to learn and adopt. These are really survival skills—and it's never too early to start.

Often, I take an inventory of what my patients are eating, where they're eating, and what triggers deterioration into binging on junk food. Usually, they say the problem is that they're busy: Their kids are in a lot of activities, and they want to show up at those activities to be supportive. On the nights when the kids have soccer, dance, music, or whatever lessons, parents make the conscious decision to reprioritize. That usually means forgoing the home-cooked meal for the sake of a drive-through meal, picking up takeout, or ordering a pizza. Instead, with just a little forethought, they could thaw out a home-cooked meal frozen a day or two earlier or even eat planned leftovers from the night before. Since these are not, typically, once-a-month situations, planning ahead for the meal at home (instead of takeout) could become a regular thing. But it's tough when everyone else on the team is piling into the car after practice and heading to the local pizzeria. That's where parents have to stand firm instead of giving in and supporting bad habits. I fully endorse the need for parents to be present for their children and their numerous after-school activities. Deciding to show up for these activities makes sense, but it should not be at the expense of their children's nutritional well-being. As important as these activities are, nutrition still takes top priority. Despite how much you want your children to succeed, they will be far less successful if, in their teens, they are battling obesity, prediabetes, fatty liver, and the early stages of heart disease.

Developing a healthy environment for kids includes limiting TV time—no more than one hour per day. And that one hour of screen time shouldn't be when preparing or eating meals.

Perhaps most importantly, a healthy environment includes a sense of mindfulness. That involves scheduling a quiet time, eliminating distractions, to think about life and talk with the children.

Mindfulness in the kitchen is also important. When preparing the meal, mom and dad need to converse with the kids—ask about their day, ask about school, ask about plans and goals. Through mindfulness and conversation, meals are transformed from being more than just a box checked off the day's to-do list. Some of my fondest memories, both growing up and as an adult, were serious conversations I had with my mother and father in the kitchen while we were all preparing a meal. It's benefit simply won't go out of style.

As a physician, I've seen too many patients with fatty liver and metabolic syndrome who are tremendously deficient in their understanding of nutrition and health, food shopping, vegetable and fruit selection, and how to prepare meals in a sustainable way. By "sustainable," I mean the cook should be creative and not just boil chicken every night. That's not sustainable. Who wouldn't get sick of boiled chicken seven days a week for a month? I would. I'd be the first to go out and get a pepperoni pizza.

# It's a National Problem

I propose that at the national level we start to own the problem. Resolving the issue of a nutrition and health deficit must be a priority for the nation. The issues of obesity and metabolic syndrome do not bode well for future generations. Today's kids are going to have a miserable existence if we don't begin to turn the tide. Obesity and all of its associated complications is enough to not only bankrupt our healthcare system but also destroy our economy. In twenty years, the typical American worker will be obese with diabetes and heart disease, popping fifteen pills each day, and spending more time in the doctor's office than at work.

One way to turn the tide, as mentioned in chapter two, would be to reinstate education along the lines of home economics. That term may be polarizing today, conjuring up the image of an aproned woman in the kitchen, but that doesn't negate the need. Today's "home ec" is for dads, young and single men and women, and youth still in school. And it should be more about life skills—how to keep a home budget, how to shop, what nutritional eating is all about, how to prepare nutritious meals. Again, people are not born knowing how to cook, clean, and manage a home, and these skills are not unique to females.

Having organized classes in school, from grade school through college level, could enhance learning at home. In college, one of my nutrition classes had a "lab" in the kitchen where we learned the theory of cooking. Those lessons remain with me today.

Since teachers in schools have a tremendous influence over children, life skills in nutrition, cooking, and meal preparation could become an extension of the classroom, helping parents and siblings become a supportive network to train students and create some excitement about these subjects.

There could even be community-based nutrition boot camps where neighborhoods or groups organize immersive and intensive two-, four-, or six-week programs to really get people up to speed. Perhaps there could even be collaborations with food manufacturers, kitchen appliance and gadget makers, grocery stores, hospitals, and other health facilities for some sort of graduation at the end of the program. Participants could be recognized for having met the learning objectives of understanding obesity and metabolic disease, the ins and outs of grocery shopping, food safety and meal preparation, and planning a tasteful series of meals that their family won't reject after a week. All of these activities should be done in the spirit of wanting to create a health environment for our families.

An expanded knowledge of nutrition must be programmed early. Even very young children can wash vegetables and learn to measure ingredients. As they get older, they can start learning to use knives to chop up vegetables and fruits, mix ingredients together, using some of the electric gadgets in the kitchen, or even cook over the stove. Of course, safety is of utmost importance, so supervision will be key as they get more involved in kitchen activities.

That's where fathers, mothers, and grandparents, and other adults and caregivers must get involved—at home, at school, and in the community. The better children understand health and nutrition, the more they make the connection that too much screen time, poor food choices, and lack of exercise lead to being overweight. Again, there are ramifications and long-term complications of children not having a better understanding of health and nutrition.

# Evolving the Picky Palate

Remember, it comes down to understanding deceptive tactics when it comes to food. Consider these foods that appear to be better choices, but in reality are not:

**Protein bars.** These may actually have good-for-you ingredients such as oatmeal, almonds, or honey, but many of them are candy bars in disguise, loaded with fat, sugar, and calories.

**Veggie chips.** Even if a chip is touted as being made of zucchini or beets or another healthy vegetable, it's still deep fried and loaded with salt.

**Margarine.** While often touted as a low-fat alternative to butter, margarine is man-made and loaded with chemicals. In the long run, butter—used sparingly—is actually a better choice.

**Rice cakes.** They're light and with few calories, but they're also made from carbs that digest quickly and cause you to crave more food.

**Bottled fruit juices and energy drinks.** These products are flavored sugar water in a bottle. Some of them contain electrolytes or other replenishing ingredients, suitable for athletes after a tough workout, but not for sedentary kids and adults.

**Multigrain, or "heart-healthy" whole wheat breads.** The grains in these breads can be similar to those in white bread, which can raise insulin levels and lead to stored belly fat. A better choice is whole grain, which contains fiber and antioxidants.

**Kid-friendly foods.** Far too often, food marketed to kids contains some of the worst ingredients. They're heavily laden with sugar, fat, or other unhealthy ingredients, and emblazoned with colorful, cartooned labels designed to entice kids. Take kids' yogurt, for instance. Even if the label screams "non-GMO" or "contains vitamin D," sprinkling candies or crumbled cookies on top pretty much negates what otherwise might be somewhat of a healthy choice.

The problem with many kid-friendly foods is that parents often give in to the gimmicks to appease a child's picky palate. Unfortunately, that gets children accustomed to eating only supersweet, supersalty, artificially flavored foods that explode in the mouth and set off a reaction in the brain. All those treats just adulterate children's taste buds, creating the problem in the first place. Following that up with a piece of cauliflower is doomed to fail; children are sure to spit it out because their brain has, in a sense, adapted to a different way of eating.

When it comes to dealing with picky eaters, first and foremost, be patient, because people go through various phases of pickiness. Here are some strategies to help deal with a child who picks and chooses what to eat:

- ✓ Have at least one item on the child's plate that you know the child likes.

- ✓ Introduce different flavors, even some that the child may not like.

- ✓ Have a variety of colorful foods on the plate.

- ✓ Get creative with food combinations. Change sizes, shapes, and consistency to make food more appealing.

- ✓ Make trying new foods a family sport.

- ✓ Involve the kids in shopping and have them help make a grocery list that is healthy.

- ✓ Don't bring unhealthy food choices home. That way, the only choice for a snack is nuts or an apple, instead of chips, cookies, or candy.

- ✓ Have set times for snacks and make them healthy choices.

- ✓ Do not reward good eating with unhealthy snacks. They caused the problem in the first place—no cookies as a reward for eating broccoli.

- ✓ Don't overwhelm the child by forcing him or her to eat everything on the plate. That can promote a bad habit of overeating. A bite or two of unpopular foods can help alter their palate to healthier choices over time.

- ✓ Try using spices and herbs. Just as adults do, kids can develop a taste for a favorite flavor and want it on everything. Look for low-sodium and salt-free options.

- ✓ Eat without distractions—no TV while at the dinner table. Meal time should be a time to slow down and talk to each other.

- ✓ Never give up. Just because a child picked over a food one time doesn't mean that child will do it again.

Above all, remember that the competition are those hyperflavored, hyped foods that have tainted the child's taste buds. Don't give the competition an edge by giving in. Kids are very manipulative, and it's up to parents to avoid giving in to their very primitive reactions. Avoid getting into a battle over food; being understanding and supportive will gain more ground than being punitive. With a little effort, and by never giving up, the competition can be overcome.

Changing a lifestyle, especially when it comes to nutrition these days, is more than uphill; it's up-mountain. But by creating a supportive environment, and lovingly standing your ground, sooner or later you will succeed. There really is no alternative.

## Meal Planning: The Best Strategy for Healthier Eating

The best strategy for combating poor eating habits is planning ahead. In the last chapter, I discussed having a plan for shopping. To recap, when planning for a trip to the grocery store: create a plan for several meals, have a detailed shopping list, never go grocery shopping when you're hungry, skip all those tempting free samples, and minimize the number of times you shop.

First on the list before shopping is creating a multiday menu. That means planning out the meals for a few days or an entire week. Here are a few basic tips to get you started.

- ✓ Consider the week's activities. This can help determine how much time you have to prepare meals.
- ✓ Map out the meals for each week and how many people need to be fed.

- ✓ Check the refrigerator, freezer, and pantry for foods already on hand to help with some of the meal decisions.

- ✓ Determine what foods can be made and eaten over several days. For instance, if you make a roast on Sunday, can the leftovers be made into Monday lunchbox meals?

- ✓ Locate any needed recipes, and determine which ingredients are common to these recipes. Some components of recipes can even be used for other meals during the week, or frozen and used later. For instance, a basic homemade tomato sauce recipe can be served on pasta one night and used with sautéed vegetables the next.

- ✓ Start a shopping list based on the meals. Be sure to include all ingredients for the week's recipes. Again, check the refrigerator, freezer, and pantry to ensure all ingredients are on the list.

At my practice, we share with patients a twenty-one-day meal plan. Go to www.drjoegalati.com for more on this meal plan and other healthy eating ideas.

Remember that meal planning, preparation, and eating should be joyful. It should never be just a box to be checked off, a routine like taking out the garbage or paying bills. There has to be a good feeling that the food being created is something your family will enjoy, but also is good for them today, tomorrow, and in the future. You have to realize *preparing these healthful meals is a gift for your family and their well-being.* Eating is a source of nutrition for the body, not just to satisfy hunger pangs.

## Kitchen Staples

You don't need a PhD in food science to make absolutely memorable meals. With just a few ingredients, you can make flavorful meals that will satisfy the entire family. Sometimes that means working with ingredients you have on hand. By keeping the kitchen stocked with a few staples, you can put together a meal whenever needed, helping you resist the impulse to order takeout. Here are some basics ingredients with which to stock a healthy kitchen.

- ✓ beans, rice, pasta, oatmeal, and whole-grain breads
- ✓ onions
- ✓ fresh spinach and romaine lettuce
- ✓ canned tomatoes and frozen vegetables
- ✓ fresh peanut or almond butter
- ✓ olive oil and vinegars (red and white wine and balsamic)
- ✓ herbs and spices such as parsley, basil, rosemary, garlic powder, cinnamon, chili powder, turmeric, oregano, nutmeg, crushed red pepper, paprika.
- ✓ reduced-fat milk and plain Greek yogurt
- ✓ eggs
- ✓ butter
- ✓ meats (frozen or fresh): Chicken or turkey and fish such as salmon or cod

# Bring Back the Dinner Party

I believe passionately that cooking and eating together should not only be a team sport for the immediate family but also a chance to connect with friends, neighbors, extended family, and even coworkers. It's a chance for people to catch up and forget about work, forget about their troubles (or maybe talk about their troubles) while breaking bread. There's something very magical about coming together around food with the chance to tell stories, share experiences, and learn from one another. This was the essence of my life growing up in New York with my family.

To do that, I'm a big advocate of bringing back the dinner party. Dinner parties are not only a feast of food, but a feast of friendship. By feast, I don't mean a table laden with so many complicated recipes that it takes weeks to plan and prepare. In fact, historically, potlucks tend to be a lot of less-than-healthful menu selections brought together. Instead, a dinner party can be composed of very simple dishes. Just getting together is something most people think is pretty special, pretty memorable. It's not about how expensive the beef filet was; it is about the energy people share with each other.

Dinner parties can even be a way to get more people interested in nutrition and cooking a healthful meal, and caring about one another. It's one thing for everyone to meet at a restaurant for dinner. But preparing a meal together is another level of engagement. And again, it's a good role model for the children to see mom and dad and other adults preparing food together. That energy and excitement can rub off on the younger generations.

Even if the thought of cooking in front of someone else seems intimidating, there are a lot of simple recipes with just a handful of ingredients that a novice would feel comfortable putting together. And most people are pretty forgiving if a recipe doesn't turn out exactly as planned. That trial and error is all part of the fun and learning process.

Making dinner a rotational event, taking place monthly at different homes, can encourage others to get involved. Over time, as others get more comfortable participating in the activity, more people will learn about nutrition—and teach others.

## The Great American Produce Giveaway

Throughout my thirty years of practicing medicine, I have found that many of my patients know very little about vegetables and fruits, and often they are intimidated by how to prepare and eat them. In fact, many are confused by the various choices; they really don't know the difference between a squash, an eggplant or peppers.

Over time, I started sharing with patients more information about various foods, including how to cook and serve them to their families. I even began bringing vegetables to the office as visual aids, and I'd share favorite, easy recipes to get them started. In time, the efforts began to work. Patients would come back months later sharing how the recipes had evolved, and how their nutrition habits had improved. Not only were my patients cooking better foods but their family, including grandchildren, were becoming energized with these new food activities.

Ultimately, these efforts evolved into what we now call the Great American Produce Giveaway. Through the giveaway, I bring in baskets of vegetables and some fruits to share with patients, along with instructions and simple recipes for preparing them. Whenever a patient is struggling to understand good nutrition, my staff will grab a bag of veggies and a recipe to give them, and they will share instructions to help get them started. We then share the activity on social media, and ask the patients to also report their results for us to share. Often, they send us a video of themselves cooking and eating the food. There is a discernible smile on their faces, and they feel good about themselves. This effort has made a major impact in their life.

To learn more about the Great American Produce Giveaway and see some patient successes, go to www.drjoegalati.com.

## It's Time to Get Real

People are coming to see me in droves with yet-to-be-diagnosed fatty liver disease. They are walking around with elevated liver chemistries, with borderline diabetes or prediabetes, with gradual weight gain that nobody is really paying attention to. Pediatric and adolescent medicine practitioners are inundated with obese children and adolescents. Yet there is an artificially established political correctness when it comes to helping patients. No patients like to be told they're overweight, even if it's coming from their physician. Physicians may tell patients they are obese, but unfortunately, recent research tells us that the conversation often ends there—no explanation, no suggestions, and no direction. Physicians are afraid of alienating their patients and the family by telling them about their weight problems. They're concerned about losing patients because the frank conversation that needs to take place may be taken the wrong way.

That is yielding to silence about an overwhelming public health crisis on the worldwide stage. I refuse to sit still and watch this happen.

It's time to get real. It's time to face the fact that if a physician is talking to you about you or a family member who is overweight and obese, it is because that physician cares. If that physician is talking to you about your child, it's because he or she realizes that your child is set up for failure. Parents have great aspirations for their children. They want them to be successful. But at this rate, in today's environment, kids are doomed. Period.

It's time to face up to the fact that it's about more than just the child. It's about the behaviors of parents, the family, the community. Junk food does not miraculously show up in your pantry. Somebody made a conscious decision to buy those Twinkies, those chips—and that's usually the parent, the one with the money in the household. It's time to begin incorporating into your life the measures I'm outlining in this book. Because, as a society, we are absolutely running out of time.

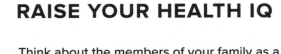

# RAISE YOUR HEALTH IQ

1.  Think about the members of your family as a cooking team. What roles would each member of the team take in preparing a meal?

2.  Take an inventory of your refrigerator, freezer, and kitchen pantry. If you had to put together a meal unexpectedly, would you have the ingredients you need?

3.  Create a one-day meal plan. Think about the day's activities, each person who needs to eat, potential recipes, and who will do what in preparing the meal.

4.  Name three friends or neighbors you would invite to a dinner party.

# CHAPTER 8

# A Few Cooking Basics

→ *Stocking the Kitchen*
→ *Getting Organized*
→ *Cooking Basics*

**Every Thursday at** noon, I'm part of a medical review board that meets as a team to systematically evaluate patients who are being considered for a liver transplant. That team effort ensures fairness for the patients being evaluated and considered for a transplant. In that evaluation, we determine the patient's suitability for a transplant, from medical, surgical, financial, and social standpoints.

Over the years, I've noticed the team has become a little bit more lax on obesity and weight limits for transplant, a direct consequence of the obesity epidemic. There's no doubt that in the current year, we are performing transplants on more obese patients than we did fifteen or twenty years ago.

One case in particular has stuck with me. It involved a patient who was significantly overweight and was not following a healthy diet. Some on the team recommended putting him on a nutrition and weight loss contract to see if he could abstain from eating junk food to potentially lose up to twenty pounds. The general consensus was that the patient would continue to overeat leading up to, and certainly after, the liver transplant, which could have serious consequences. One member of the team even stood up for the patient, asking, "Do you all realize how difficult losing weight is? Do you understand that in the setting of a chronic illness, like cirrhosis, they're not going to be able to lose weight?"

While I agree with him that it is difficult for sick people to start to eat better food and lose weight, at the same time I know it's time for us in the healthcare profession to work with patients to help them understand better eating and to give them the tools they need to take care of themselves today, before we get to an end-stage organ failure situation.

That's one reason I've included this chapter about some kitchen basics. I'd be remiss if I didn't comment on the kitchen and cooking. An operational kitchen, where basic meals can be prepared, is a prerequisite to a healthy lifestyle. I believe people really do want to get back to the basics, but many of them just don't know how.

When it comes to cooking, it's important to feel comfortable making modest meals before launching into complicated recipes. Beginner cooks need to know how to make simple meals that are nutritious and tasty and will keep everybody's attention. There are many ways to incorporate vegetables and proteins into a good diet that anyone can enjoy. These cooking skills need to be discussed.

## Stocking the Kitchen

There is nothing worse than trying to cook a meal at home and not having the necessary ingredients. This is probably the number-one reason patients tell me they don't cook at home: an ill-supplied kitchen. The refrigerator is filled with moldy cheese, stale lunch-meats, wilted greens, and a few sparse pieces of fruit. The freezer has food that's outdated and should be tossed. The shelves of your pantry have a jar of Cheez Whiz, a box of mac and cheese, and pretzels. This is not a scenario that can produce a healthful meal for you and the family.

Having just a few basics on hand makes all the difference in the world. Paying attention to the refrigerator, freezer, and pantry takes just a few minutes of thought each week. The windfall of such thinking is invaluable in the long term.

For healthier eating, there are a few foods that I recommend having on-hand all the time. These simple ingredients can help get you started learning how to get comfortable in the kitchen.

## Produce: Fruits and Vegetables

Always have a supply of fresh fruit on hand. Based on your likings, these might include strawberries, blueberries, apples, pears, various citrus fruits, and melons (in season). Obviously, these have a limited shelf life, so planning will need to include consumption of these throughout the week.[63]

Some fruits can remain at room temperature, others should be refrigerated. Generally speaking, do not wash the fruit until it's ready to be eaten or used in a dish. As you get more familiar with buying fruit, you'll be able to select fruit that is ready to eat and fruit that will ripen later in the week when you're ready to eat it.

I recommend purchasing organic fruits and vegetables, which tend to have less residue of pesticides, reducing your exposure to possible toxins and negative health effects. These include:

- ✓ strawberries
- ✓ apples
- ✓ nectarines
- ✓ peaches
- ✓ celery
- ✓ grapes
- ✓ cherries
- ✓ spinach
- ✓ tomatoes
- ✓ bell peppers
- ✓ cucumbers

As with fruit, try to plan your vegetable purchases according to your weekly menu and have a variety of fresh produce on hand. While string beans and cauliflower may be your go-to vegetables, experiment with squash, zucchini, eggplant, and peppers. Search online for recipes that use all of these in combination, or recipes that may make use of just one or two of them. Visit www.drjoegalati.com for many of my favorite recipes.

Also select several greens for the week: romaine or Boston lettuce, spinach, arugula, kale, and/or fennel. Iceberg lettuce, the go-to salad starter for most, has no nutritional value; it's mostly water and has few health benefits. Avoid this nutrition-poor product.

When tossing together a salad, remember that commercially made salad dressings tend to be high in salt, fat, sugar, and calories, as do croutons. Avoid any dressing labeled as "creamy." Instead, consider using olive oil with a couple tablespoons of balsamic vinegar and maybe a few of your favorite herbs and spices for a little bit of added punch.

## Storing Fresh Fruits and Vegetables for Best Flavor

### Store in the refrigerator

| Fruit: | Vegetables: |
|---|---|
| Apples (more than 7 days), Apricots, Asian pears, Berries, Cherries, Cut Fruit, Figs, Grapes | Artichokes, Asparagus, Green Beans, Beets, Belgian Endive, Broccoli, Brussel Sprouts, Cabbage, Carrots, Cauliflower, Celery, Cut Vegetables, Green Onions, Herbs (not basil), Leafy Vegetables, Leeks, Lettuce, Mushrooms, Peas, Radishes, Spinach, Sprouts, Summer Squashes, Sweet Corn |

### Ripen on the counter first

Avocados, Kiwi, Nectarines, Peaches, Pears, Plums, Plumcots

### Ripen on the counter

| Fruit: | Vegetables: |
|---|---|
| Apples, (fewer than 7 days), Bananas, Citrus fruits, Mangoes, Melons, Papayas, Persimmons, Pineapple, Plantain, Pomegranates | Basil (in water), Cucumber[†], Eggplant[†], Garlic, Ginger, Jicama, Onions, Peppers, Potatoes, Pumpkins, Sweet Potatoes, Tomatoes, Winter Squashes |

Source: https://www.fruitsandveggiesmorematters.org/wp-content/uploads/UserFiles/File/pdf/why/Storing_Fruits_Veggies_FINAL.pdf

## Dairy: Yogurt, Milk, Eggs

I like to keep Greek yogurt on hand. Instead of a flavored variety, I like to add my own fruit (sliced apple, grapes, strawberries) to plain yogurt, which can cut down on the sugar and associated calories. Top it off with a drizzle of fresh local honey for added sweetness. Greek yogurt, typically, is an acquired taste, but after a few containers, I'm sure you'll love it. One benefit of Greek yogurt is the higher protein content, which is about twice as much as in other types of yogurt.

Organic milk is good to keep on hand. Two additives—recombinant bovine growth hormone (rBGH, also known as BGH; recombinant bovine somatotropin, or rBST) and antibiotics—are found in non-organic milk but not in organic milk. If you have an allergy to milk, then another good option is almond milk. Unsweetened almond milk with no artificial flavors has only 40 calories per serving. Almond milk works well on cereal and in smoothies. The controversy regarding cow's milk persists. Lactose intolerance is pervasive throughout the population and there are those that feel cows milk is deleterious to one's health, contributing to heart disease, obesity, and cancer.

A variety of cheeses, such as fresh mozzarella or imported cheddars, can be used sparingly on eggs, in salads, or with other dishes. If you are on a salt-restricted diet, look for low-salt varieties. Beware of cottage cheese, touted as a diet staple. It is loaded with salt.

| Sodium in Cheese—An Eye Opener Sodium/mg/serving | | | |
|---|---|---|---|
| Cheddar Cheese: 174 | Gouda: 232 | Romano: 340 | American: 368 |
| Blue cheese: 395 | Parmesan: 454 | Cottage cheese: 819 | |

Eggs are also considered to be dairy. Eggs are a tremendous source of protein and nutrients. The concern about cholesterol in eggs is far less controversial than it was fifteen years ago, so consider consuming an egg three or four days per week. Eggs are essential for cooking. Once you master a scrambled egg, and then an omelet, the possibilities for meals are endless. Omelets can be made with leftover chicken, beef, or even fish and/or chopped veggies, or a sliver of cheese. Pure egg whites are a good option for keeping eggs in the house. Make sure the container says 100 percent liquid egg whites. At 25 calories and 5 grams of protein per serving, these are exceptional additions to any egg dish. I like to use one whole egg and mix the equivalent of two or three additional egg whites in my mixing bowl when I make an omelet.

Also keep fresh butter on hand but use it sparingly. Skip the margarine, which is loaded with chemicals. Remember it's a man food.

## Protein: Meats, Fish, And Nuts

When it comes to ground beef, you're better off purchasing it at a market that grinds it fresh daily. The quality and risk of a food-borne illness is just too high with mass-produced, premanufactured ground beef. You may even want to purchase a meat grinder and grind your own meats at home. There are many ways of using lean ground beef, chicken, or turkey in your menus. However, most prefer their red meat in the form of steak. Small 4 oz. filets are best for health and weight-conscious cooks. There is rather convincing evidence that excessive red meat is associated with colon cancer, so it may best to go sparingly with red meat and lean more toward chicken, turkey, and higher-quality cuts of pork, of course avoiding sausage, bacon, and other processed meats. *Let me reiterate that meat consumption needs to be done with extreme moderation. My goal is to support a mostly plant-based diet.*

Also keep tuna fish and pink salmon on hand. These are excellent sources of protein and vitamins in a low-fat food.

Whenever possible, have on hand salt-free, raw varieties of nuts. These versions have no oil and fewer calories. Eat a few as a snack, incorporate them into a smoothie, or add them to a vegetable dish.

## Prepared Foods

Avoid prepackaged, frozen foods. Frozen dinners and premade meals may seem convenient, but you're going to pay for it in the end with a meal that does not contribute to good health. The only acceptable items from the frozen section are vegetables and fruits—and *only* those—nothing with added cheese, salt, seasonings, or sugar. Growing up, Mom always had Green Giant frozen vegetables on hand for select recipes. Today, Green Giant has over 175 products to choose from. As discussed earlier in this book, this overwhelming selection leads to consumer confusion and poor choices. If you're buying frozen lima beans, the only ingredient in the bag should be lima beans. Frozen fruits are ideal to keep on hand for smoothies, snacks, desserts, and salads.

Also avoid keeping on hand snacks such as chips, candy, soda, and artificially sweetened and colored drinks. If you buy them and they enter your house, you're going to eat them. Make your home a chip-soda-candy-snack free zone.

A quick word about your favorite deli meats. Regardless of the advertising hype, these are heavily processed meats. A steady diet of lunchmeats needs to be avoided because research suggests these meats are filled with carcinogens and increase your risk of cancer. In addition to their preservatives, they are high in sodium. Looking carefully at the label, a serving is 2 oz. of meat. As a former New York Italian deli man, that is one skimpy sandwich! A typical sandwich is 4 oz. of sliced meat, which will double the sodium content. So while 2 oz. of beef bologna has 540 mg of sodium, a standard sandwich has double, or a whopping 1,080 mg, keeping in mind the daily limit should be around 1500 for the day. Add a piece or two of cheese on your sandwich, and you have met your sodium target for the day.

There are only a few acceptable canned goods to keep on hand. A variety of beans, for instance, but these should be rinsed thoroughly before eating or cooking. Doing so removes the excess salt used in packing, yet retains the fiber and nutrients that are present in these little wonders. Canned beans can be used as a side dish, incorporated into salads, or combined with other vegetables or rice. They are filling, low in calories, and great from a nutritional standpoint. Once you acquire the taste of canned beans, experiment cooking a batch of fresh bean from scratch. The added effort will reward you with a nutritionally awesome meal.

Pasta and noodles are also okay in limited quantities. These can be incorporated into your meals on occasion.

### A Word about Fiber

Whenever possible, add fiber to your menu, thirty-five to forty grams a day. While adding raw vegetables and fruit to a salad—onions, radishes, apples, avocado—can certainly add fiber to a salad, the real winner in the high fiber arena is legumes. Black beans, kidney beans, garbanzo beans—incorporate them into lunch and dinner and you'll be getting plenty of fiber—fifteen grams per serving.

Contrary to popular belief, multigrain bran muffins are not the best way to go when it comes to fiber (people love to brag that they eat bran muffins for their daily fiber!). Again, these can raise insulin levels and lead to unhealthy fat storage. Similarly, bran cereals only have five grams of fiber. Even Metamucil, a leading soluble-fiber supplement, only has three grams of dietary fiber and two grams of soluble fiber in a single tablespoon serving. Add to that the other ingredients—eight grams of sugar plus sucrose, citric acid, natural and artificial orange flavor, and yellow dye number 6—and you're much better off eating a serving of beans. Trust me, a scoopful of Metamucil in a glass is not going to be as satisfying as a cup of beans prepared with your favorite seasonings. Plus, you're getting all the phytonutrients with antioxidant and anti-inflammatory properties that are supporting good health. Go to www.drjoegalati.com for more tips on fiber.

| World's Healthiest Foods Rich in Fiber | | | |
|---|---|---|---|
| Food | Calories per serving | Grams of fiber per serving | % of Daily Requirement per serving |
| Navy Beans | 255 | 19 | 76% |
| Dried Peas | 231 | 16 | 65% |
| Lentils | 230 | 16 | 63% |
| Pinto Beans | 245 | 15 | 62% |
| Black Beans | 227 | 15 | 60% |
| Lima Beans | 216 | 13 | 53% |
| Garbanzo Beans | 269 | 12 | 50% |
| Tempeh | 222 | 12 | 48% |
| Kidney Beans | 225 | 11 | 45% |
| Barley | 217 | 11 | 42% |

Source: http://whfoods.org/genpage.php?tname=nutrient&dbid=59#deficiencysymptoms

## Learn to Love Oatmeal

Always have a supply of oatmeal in the house. While Quaker Oats (old-fashioned) is a good choice, Quaker Quick 1-Minute Oats are also acceptable. This version is not chemically altered, just put through a press to allow it to cook quicker and absorb water faster. Avoid instant microwave and flavored oat meals, which only add more calories, chemicals, and artificial sweeteners to your precious body.

## Spices and Herbs

As I mentioned in the previous chapter, spices and herbs can flavor a dish without adding salt. They're a great, inexpensive way to experiment as you become more comfortable in the kitchen. Plus, they're an excellent alternative to salt. Some of my favorites are basal, garlic, rosemary, pepper, thyme, basil, chive, oregano, chili powder, bay leaf, cinnamon, ginger, mustard, paprika, nutmeg, and parsley. The key is to have the freedom to experiment, have fun in the kitchen, and enjoy trying to make flavorful food. A draw containing six to eight spices and herbs is a good start for you.

## Special Note about Salt Substitutes

These have potassium chloride as the salt, as opposed to sodium chloride (table salt). If you have heart, kidney, or liver disease, or you're on certain medications, you can develop a toxic level of potassium, which can be fatal. Look for salt-free blends such as Mrs. Dash. Many people with kidney problems are unable to eliminate excessive potassium, which could result in a deadly cardiac complication. The safest approach is to simply avoid these products.

Anyone interested in cooking needs some basic information. The rest of the chapter covers some of those basics. But I encourage you to learn more by sharing with others, researching online or in bookstores, or checking out my website at www.drjoegalati.com.

## Getting Organized

Cooking at home requires a bit of organization. No one likes to get halfway through a recipe only to discover that an ingredient is missing. That means having on hand the ingredients for a recipe, and also having all the tools and utensils needed to complete all the steps in the recipe.

Here are some of the items you'll need to equip your kitchen before starting to cook.

### Knives

These are probably the most important tools in the kitchen. I'd avoid spending the money on a full knife set in a block. Instead, start with three that will allow you to do 95 percent of the cutting required.

There are three knives to start off with in any kitchen:

A utility knife, sometimes known as a paring knife, is used for peeling and cutting smaller vegetables and cuts of meat, when you don't quite need an eight-inch chef's knife. Three- or four-inch paring knives can be purchased for $10 to $35.

A serrated-edge knife, which has a saw-tooth edge, is handy for cutting tomatoes, vegetables, fruits, melons, fatty cuts of meat, or for slicing bread.

An easy-to-handle chef's knife with a blade from six to eight inches long is a good tool for slicing and chopping. Spending $35 can get you a good-quality chef's knife.

Use the right knife for the job, and ensure it is sharp; dull knives can slip more easily. Hold the knife handle firmly, and when chopping or dicing, keep the tip of the blade on or close to the cutting board.

## Cutting Boards

It's best to have two cutting boards, one for meats, and another for veggies, herbs, and all other foods. Segregating the cutting boards can help eliminate the spread of harmful bacteria from raw meat to other foods that are not cooked.

## Cooking Pots, Pans, and Bake Ware

Your basic kitchen toolset should include

- ✓ 8-quart stockpot with lid
- ✓ 2- and 4-quart saucepans with lids
- ✓ 8- to 10-inch frying pan
- ✓ 14 x 18-inch rimmed cookie sheet
- ✓ A large baking dish (casserole)

The stockpot with lid and saucepans with lids are for cooking and heating up foods.

A good frying pan can be one of the handiest tools you'll have. Use it to cook everything from eggs, to vegetables, to meats, to one-skillet meals. While some people opt for a Teflon nonstick surface, remember these scratch easily. Other options include stainless steel, which are one of the most durable choices, or cast iron, also durable but requires seasoning before use.

A 14 x 18-inch cookie sheet is also a good to have on hand, ideal for roasting vegetables.

One large and one medium-size mixing bowl should handle your entire novice cooking needs.

Glass Pyrex dishes with lids let you cook and refrigerate food in the same container.

## A Variety of Utensils and Kitchen Gadgets

These should include the following:

- ✓ a box grater for shredding vegetables, cheese, and fruits
- ✓ spatula (heat resistant) for scraping the sides of bowls or pans
- ✓ measuring spoons: a set should include at least a half teaspoon, a teaspoon, and a tablespoon
- ✓ measuring cups with clearly marked measures on the side
- ✓ mixing spoons: a couple of large, long-handled wooden or heat-resistant spoons
- ✓ vegetable peeler for taking the skins off vegetables
- ✓ meat thermometer for ensuring meat is cooked to the right temperature
- ✓ colander for draining cooked vegetables and washing fruit

- ✓ potato masher for mashing cooked potatoes and other cooked vegetables

- ✓ garlic press for crushing garlic cloves

- ✓ oven mitts or potholders for handling hot pots and pans

- ✓ trivets for placing hot pans on a tabletop

- ✓ vegetable spiralizer to make a healthy alternative to regular pasta

Once your kitchen is equipped, it's time to get cooking. Let's look at a few cooking basics.

## Cooking Basics

With a little practice, you can gain the confidence you need to put together meals on a daily basis. To get started, consider these cooking basics.

### Food Safety

As you learn to cook with fresh foods, you'll need to know how to store them. Fresh foods have a shorter lifespan, so here again, planning and organization are important. For more in-depth information, check with your local extension office for a food handlers class. Many states offer a course online for a nominal fee.

In the meantime, here are some quick tips:

**Freezer storage times**

- ✓ steaks: 6–12 months

- ✓ chops: 4–6 months

- ✓ bacon: 1 month

- ✓ seafood: 2 months

- ✓ whole chicken: 1 month

**Refrigerator storage times**

- ✓ luncheon meat: 3–5 days (opened); 2 weeks (unopened)

- ✓ bacon: 7 days

- ✓ hamburger and sausage, raw: 1–2 days

- ✓ beef and pork steaks, chops, and roasts: 3–5 days

- ✓ fresh poultry: 1–2 days

- ✓ leftovers: 3–4 days

Cross-contamination is an issue when dealing with raw and cooked foods. Raw foods should always be kept on a plate or in a tray to catch any potential spillage. Store foods with enough room around them for air to circulate. Keep vegetables and fruits in separate drawers. Store dairy and eggs on higher shelves, above cooked foods or leftovers.

## Cutting Fat from Your Meal/Diet

Although a certain amount of fat is to be expected in foods, there are some simple ways to trim the fat while cooking.

- ✓ Start by removing visible fat from meats, and remove the skin from poultry.

- ✓ Drain browned beef after cooking; you can even blot away fats with paper towels.

- ✓ With a spoon, skim excess fat off meat sauces, chili, and stew or chill these dishes and then remove the hardened fat.

- ✓ Use a minimal amount of olive oil or butter when cooking, or use a nonstick pan, which may require no oil.

- ✓ Opt for low-fat methods of cooking such as roasting, baking, grilling, stir-frying, broiling, or boiling.

## Working with Vegetables

Size matters when eating vegetables. For instance, when eating raw vegetables in a salad or as a snack, cut them into smaller pieces. When cooking vegetables, cut them into similar shapes and sizes to promote cooking at roughly the same rate.

Some vegetables are commonly peeled before eating, including turnips, potatoes, carrots, and cucumbers. But some people prefer to leave the peel on since a lot of nutrients and fiber are in it.

## Portion Size

Learning to cook also means controlling portion size. You need to know how much food to make, depending on the number of people you're feeding. Here are some per-person guidelines:

- ✓ 4 oz. meat, fish, or poultry are about the size of two decks of playing cards.

- ✓ 4 oz. vegetables

- ✓ 2 oz. beans or legumes

- ✓ 2 oz. rice or pasta as a side dish, about one-fourth cup cooked

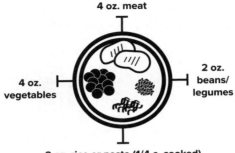

4 oz. meat

2 oz. beans/legumes

4 oz. vegetables

2 oz. rice or pasta (1/4 c. cooked)

If these numbers sound very small, remember this: Healthy food is more filling. While it may seem to be a little bit of food, these portions satisfy more than a larger quantity of junk food. We all need to recalibrate our serving size expectation. As stated earlier, over the years, portion size has gradually increased proportionally to the obesity statistics we are now facing.

## A Handy Guide to Portion Control

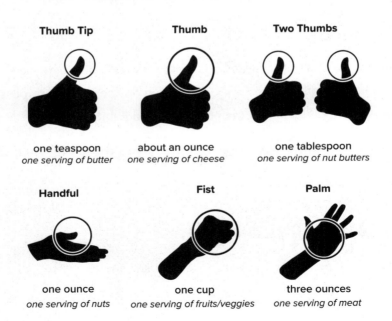

**Thumb Tip**
one teaspoon
*one serving of butter*

**Thumb**
about an ounce
*one serving of cheese*

**Two Thumbs**
one tablespoon
*one serving of nut butters*

**Handful**
one ounce
*one serving of nuts*

**Fist**
one cup
*one serving of fruits/veggies*

**Palm**
three ounces
*one serving of meat*

I'm not a certified chef. I'm a cooking enthusiast. But I think if you just follow my lead, you will eat a great diet. My hope is to enlighten you that cooking at home is the only option to reduce and turn around the rising tide of obesity and associated diseases, including fatty liver. If you take the time to learn how to cook ten different vegetable dishes, with minor variations to each, you can prevent the humdrum boredom of steamed broccoli night after night. Have four or five smoothie recipes to start your day, and learn to make an omelet using fresh eggs or egg whites and adding in a range of meats and veggies. And there are countless dishes that can be made with the basic staples of a few vegetables, chicken, fish, and beef.

The problem with so many patients is that they are told to eat more fruits and vegetables, but they don't know what fruits and vegetables to eat. They are told to eat a lower-carb diet, but they're not even sure what a carb is. Carbs, or carbohydrates, are the sugars, starches and fibers found in fruits, grains, vegetables and milk products. Carbs provide fuel for the central nervous system and energy for working muscles. Simple carbs are quickly digested and lead to sudden bursts of glucose in the blood. Examples include simple sugars like those found in certain fruits, milk, table sugar, and of course soda and candy. Complex carbs, the preferred type, are found in starchy foods including beans, peas, lentils, peanuts, potatoes, corn, parsnips, whole-grain breads and cereals.

**Complex carbs are found in starchy foods including beans, peas, lentils, peanuts, potatoes, corn, parsnips, whole-grain breads and cereals. These carbs breakdown slower and wreak less havoc on your blood sugar and insulin levels.**

These carbs breakdown slower and wreak less havoc on your blood sugar and insulin levels. They're told they eat out too much, but they don't know how to cook for themselves or others at home. There is one thing that I am very sure of: consistently eating out is a hazard to your health. You will never regain wellness with these lifestyle choices.

I hope this chapter has given you some tools to be successful. I want you to be excited about cooking. I want you to feel there's hope even though you've been given a diagnosis of fatty liver or diabetes. You and your family can turn things around. I know you can do it.

There's much more to learn about cooking. What I've included is just a bit to tempt you. In the online appendix, I've included more cooking tips and directions. And for more information, go to www.drjoegalati.com.

In the next chapter—no groaning, folks—I'll discuss exercise, another area in a changing lifestyle.

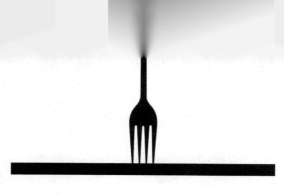

# RAISE YOUR HEALTH IQ

1.  Choose three that you think would make a good combination for a smoothie:

    • kale

    • spinach

    • fresh ginger

    • ground flaxseed

    • carrots

    • almond milk

    • beets

2.  Name three ways to cook an egg.

3.  Name three nutritious ingredients for an omelet.

4.  Name three spices or herbs you'd be inclined to buy and use.

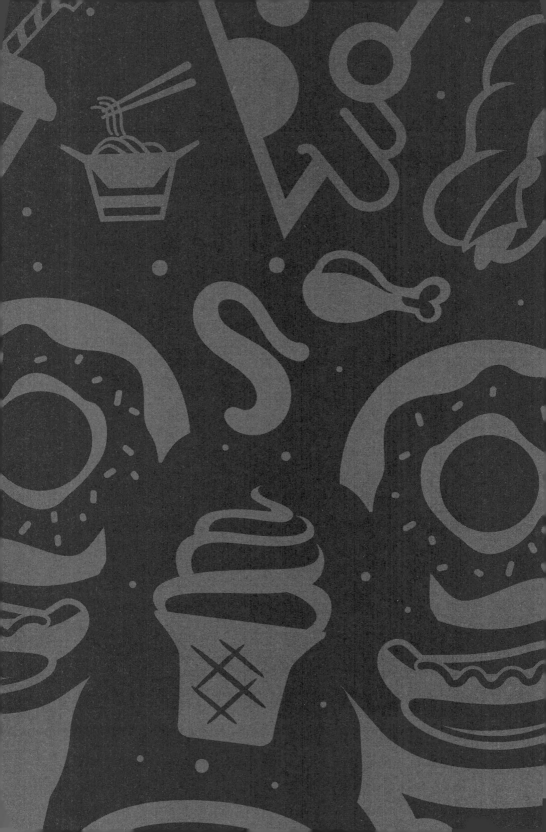

# CHAPTER 9

# Exercise: It's A Good Thing

**Sam had hepatitis** C for about twenty years before coming to see me. He had undergone two prior treatment regimens that were incredibly difficult, filled with toxic side effects. Fortunately, a third successful treatment with new and improved therapies resulted in a cure. Afterward, his life circumstances changed for the better and he ended up gaining a fair amount of weight as a result of increased business travel and eating out. Unfortunately, he also developed prediabetes and a fatty liver, which we found by accident while doing an ultrasound to follow up on his hepatitis C. Sam described the moment when he was told about his condition: "During the ultrasound, the technician leaned over and said everything looked fine except for the fact that my liver was now fatty." He was devastated.

When I confirmed Sam's diagnosis, he—and his wife—were alarmed into cleaning up their diet and beginning a regular exercise routine. After three painful therapies for hepatitis C, kicking the smoking habit, and being sober from alcohol for over twenty years, Sam declared, "Eating too much ice cream is not going to take me down." Within a year, his health had reverted back to normal following a regular exercise program and eliminating sweets and excess calories. His prediabetes was gone, and his fatty liver was no longer detected by an ultrasound. Sam is a perfect example of what happens when people take their eye off their health and experience a decline in wellness. But he's also a great example of what can happen when people are mindful of their nutrition and the value of exercise, which can make all the difference and even turn things around.

## The Role of Exercise

It's very hard to simply lose weight and maintain fitness with diet alone. Exercise combining aerobic and weight training helps improve weight loss by increasing your basal metabolic rate (the energy in calories needed to keep the body functioning while at rest), your strength, balance, and overall wellness. If you're looking to lose weight, you need to exercise.

Exercise also helps control blood sugar. It helps increase insulin sensitivity, aiding the ability of the muscles to use more of the glucose in the bloodstream. During activity, the muscles contract and the cells take up glucose to use as energy. That happens even if no insulin is available for use. Over time, that can lower blood sugar levels and make the insulin in your body work more efficiently. The human body, to remain healthy, is meant to move.

Losing weight also lowers lipids (cholesterol building blocks) and tri-glycerides, the fat in the bloodstream that, when elevated, can raise heart disease risk. In short, exercise helps control all the characters of metabolic syndrome.

Exercise also promotes smart, graceful aging by improving balance and posture, reducing the chance of dementia, and strengthening bones (reducing the risk of fractures).

I recently had a conversation with a sixty-eight-year-old patient who has had fatty liver for most of her adult life. Since she didn't eat right, exercise, lose weight, or take good care of her health, she developed cirrhosis and had finally developed a liver cancer so large that it made her ineligible for a liver transplant. As you can imagine, that was devastating news. As we discussed her care from that point forward, she asked what she could do to turn things around. "Can I eat better? Will losing weight help? What if I exercise?" she asked. I had to tell her the truth—albeit in a sensitive fashion: The reason she was in her current situation was because of twenty-five years of not eating right, not exercising, being overweight, and having poorly controlled diabetes. In short, she had not paid attention to her health for nearly half her life. At that point, eating more broccoli and cabbage wasn't going to turn things around; it wouldn't do it for her. It won't do it for anyone.

When you are in a decades-long wrestling match with aging and health and about to be thrown to the mat, you cannot think that something you do today is going to miraculously fix what hasn't been done for most of your adult life. It's heartbreaking for me to have tell patients that they've waited too long. I would love nothing more than to be able to tell people to eat cauliflower and zucchini for a year and everything will be fine. But it just doesn't work that way. The key is to intervene now—before it is too late. Wellness is a lifelong strategy, not something you pay attention to in the eleventh hour.

## Be Realistic

Especially if you have done nothing in the way of exercise for the better part of five years or longer, it's going to take time to get a regular routine. It's a good idea to get clearance from a physician before initiating a regular workout routine.

Then, to keep from getting frustrated, start out slowly and have realistic goals. Start by setting aside a portion of your day to simple activities just to begin developing a routine. Even if all you do is walk for ten minutes a day, your body will love you for taking the initiative to move, instead of sitting in an office chair all day and then coming home and lying on the couch.

Too often, people who have put off exercising and then decide to begin don't logically think through what it's going to take. It takes time to build up health after it has been neglected for so long, and to launch right in without the proper attire and proper medical condition can put you on the path to injury. That's how many of the best-intentioned exercise efforts get derailed. In fact, according to the US Consumer Product Safety Commission, in 2012, almost 500,000 people went to the hospital for injuries related to exercise equipment; about 32,000 were hospitalized or died of their injuries. Across the United States, about 24,000 treadmill-related injuries have taken place, and from 2003 to 2012, there were thirty reported deaths associated with treadmills.[64]

It's very easy to get bored, frustrated, and discouraged by an exercise program that involves only a daily trot on the treadmill at the gym. That may work for the short term, but most people need variety. Keeping exercise fresh through a variety of activities increases interest, keeps you stay motivated, and is better for your overall health. As never before, there are countless opportunities to exercise. Besides the traditional health club layout, with its treadmills and rows of free weights and exercise machines, members can participate in spin classes, yoga, Pilates, Zumba, and group exercise classes. Besides health clubs, there are dedicated facilities that specialize in kick boxing, traditional boxing, and cross-fit. There are running clubs in every town helping you train for a wide range of runs, cycle events, and walking. The message here is that with all of the opportunities to get up and move, there is no reason to simply jump on a treadmill and get bored.

## Getting Started

Whatever form of exercise you engage in, be sure to spend a few minutes warming up. A warm-up is basically a few minutes of doing the same exercise you are about to engage in, only at a slower pace. Warming up gives the various muscle groups a chance to loosen up, helping to avoid injury during a workout. It also opens the capillaries (small blood vessels), increasing blood flow from around 10 to 15 percent (while at rest) to 70 to 75 percent, which helps to improve performance during the exercise.[65]

Also consider incorporating yoga and/or tai chi into your routine. These are great ways to stay flexible and improve your core strength. With disuse, muscles have a natural tendency to tighten up and shorten, but yoga and tai chi can lengthen and strengthen muscles and improve range of motion.

Yoga is an ancient form of exercise combining stretching and movements to improve strength and flexibility and promote relaxation. Yoga movements also help lubricate the joints, ligaments, and tendons while toning muscles and improving posture. Tai chi combines deep breathing with martial arts movements to improve coordination, flexibility, and strength. Both yoga and tai chi are low-impact, weight-bearing exercises that improve balance and overall energy.

## Get Walking

One way to get started with exercise is simply by walking. Walking is a safe, low-impact exercise that most people can manage.

If you're new to exercise, start by setting a timer for a ten-minute walk. As you get more of a routine and begin to get stronger, increase the time by an extra minute or two until you're going out for thirty minutes, and then back to your stating point—a full hour walk. Be patient. It will take time to build up your endurance.

A pedometer is a useful, easy-to-use tool if walking is your exercise of choice, or to simply help you determine the amount you're moving throughout the day. The pedometer measures steps and lets you see how far you've traveled. A popular walking program is ten thousand steps, which, depending on stride length, is roughly three-and-a-half to four miles. Taking ten thousand steps a day is an important goal to work toward because research has shown that, along with other healthy habits, it can lead to a reduction in chronic illnesses such as diabetes, metabolic syndrome, and chronic heart disease. That's a very good benchmark for someone who is just starting out with exercise. Walking requires very little financial investment: All you need is a good pair of shoes and an inexpensive pedometer and you're good to go. Most smartphones today have a built-in pedometer app, or it can be purchased for a small cost.

Once you've built up a few walking muscles, measure your efforts with a heart rate monitor. The heart rate monitor can help you "get in the zone," that point in your heart rate, based on your age, at which your body burns the most fat calories. Moderate activity is about 50 to 70 percent of your maximum heart rate, and vigorous activity is 70 to 85 percent. By most reports, the fat burning range is somewhere between 60 and 70 percent of maximum. To calculate your maximum heart rate, subtract your age from 220. For example, it you're forty-five years old, your maximum heart rate is 220 − 45 = 175 beats per minute. Moderate activity would yield a target heart rate of 88 to 122 beats/minute when exercising.

There are also benefits to weight training to help increase muscle mass, build bone, and improve overall strength. A good way to incorporate a bit of weight or resistance training into a walk is to carry a set of two- to five-pound dumbbells and use them to do arm exercises as you walk. The more muscles being used, the more calories burned and the stronger and more toned you will become.

Rucking has become a popular form of exercise. Rucking involves wearing a weighted back pack while going on an extended walk. One company, GoRuck, sells durable American-made back packs (or rucksacks) designed specifically to hold weight, and it organizes rucking activities around the country. Rucking is a way to burn three times as many calories as walking while increasing muscle mass, burning more fat, improving posture, and strengthening your heart and body overall.

Hiking has always been one of my favorite activities. Hiking is essentially walking on uneven surfaces, which can make it significantly more challenging. In fact, research has shown that, compared to walking on a level surface, hiking can increase the amount of energy the body uses by nearly 30 percent.[66] Hiking requires the use of different muscles than walking, and it can up your heart rate and improve your core and balance. As with walking, it's best to start off slow with hiking, maybe taking on a shorter trail at first, since hiking comes with a few risks: it's easier to take a tumble or twist an ankle on uneven terrain. Throughout the country there are assorted organizations that offer opportunities to get involved in hiking. Contact your local chapter of the Sierra Club at www.sierraclub.org, or the outdoor retailer REI Co-op at www.rei.com for details near you.

There are also emotional and psychological benefits to being outdoors. Research has shown that being outdoors, in nature, getting a little fresh air and sunshine, lets you clear your brain, calms you down, and lets you gain some inner peace.[67] Hiking also tends to be a more social activity, one that people enjoy doing in groups, adding to the experience. So, if you really want that complete mind-body workout, think about adding a hike to your weekly exercise routine.

One other variation of walking worth a mention is alpine walking, sometimes known as Nordic walking. Basically, this involves using a pair of trekking sticks or poles while walking. Since using the poles involves the upper muscles, this type of walking helps burn more calories, contributing to more weight loss, greater fitness, and more overall strength. A good set of trekking poles can be bought for around $80 to $150.

# Aerobic Exercises

Walking, hiking, running, and dancing are all aerobic activities. Aerobic exercise is movement that gets your heart pumping, increasing blood flow to your muscles. Aerobics also make you breathe faster and deeper, increasing oxygen levels in your blood. Aerobic exercise helps remove wastes from your body, such as lactic acid and carbon dioxide, and it causes the release of endorphins, those feel-good hormones.

**The CDC recommends that adults get, in at least ten-minute increments, a weekly minimum of:**

- ✔ 2 1/2 hours of moderate-intensity aerobic activity, *or*

- ✔ 1 hour and 15 minutes of vigorous-intensity aerobic activity, *or*

- ✔ an equivalent mix of moderate- and vigorous-intensity aerobic activity.[68]

**Moderate-intensity aerobic activity includes**

- ✔ walking fast

- ✔ water aerobics

- ✔ bicycling on level or relatively level ground

- ✔ pushing a lawn mower

- ✔ vigorous house cleaning

- ✔ ballroom dancing

- ✔ low-impact aerobics

## Vigorous-intensity aerobic activity includes

- ✓ jogging or running
- ✓ hiking
- ✓ swimming laps
- ✓ bicycling fast or on hills
- ✓ playing basketball

## Strength and Resistance Training

A couple days a week, incorporate strength and resistance training into your exercise routine. As people age, they lose muscle year after year (as much as 3 to 5 percent for each decade after age thirty), a condition known as sarcopenia.[69] In young adults, strength and resistance training can increase muscle mass, tone skin, and improve bone density. In older adults, it can slow bone loss and help maintain strength.[70] Sarcopenia is the reason many older people become frail and suffer from falls and bone breaks. Strength training with weights can also reduce the risk of developing osteoporosis, or brittle bone disease, reducing the risk of a break if a fall occurs. As our population continues to age and live longer, due to all of the medical innovations they are recipients of, there are the continued issues related to muscle loss and weakness. Thought has to be given to how this is going to be addressed. It is incumbent on my physician colleagues to prescribe some type of ongoing exercise plan for their aging patients and for patients and their caretakers to take an interest in ways to keep moving and slowing down the muscle loss and muscle strength that will occur.

Weight training can be done with free weights, such as barbells, dumbbells, or hand weights. There are also ankle and wrist weights, and even weight vests that can be worn. Some of these allow for the amount of weight to be adjusted. Resistance exercises can be done with (elastic) bands that come in varying tensions, or even with your own body weight (remember pushups?). Using weight machines may be best for beginners. While accidents using these machines still occur, they are safer because they eliminate the instability that occurs when you are handling free weights. I highly recommend getting professional advice from a trainer before using these machines.

## Mix It Up

Again, variety is key. I personally get bored with exercise unless I regularly change up the type of activity that I do.

While health clubs offer a range of equipment, take care in using these. Most facilities have staff to give you at least an introduction to using the equipment properly. Don't be afraid to ask for help!

Some people find that working out with a partner or in groups helps keep them accountable, and this I highly recommend. Whether it's a good friend or a family member, or a team activity such as a group walk or workout, a basketball game, or bicycling with a club, most people are more motivated when there's a sense of responsibility to the group to show up and participate.

There is a significant movement toward high-intensity circuit training or high-intensity interval training (HIIT). And there's a fair amount of research that says you just need to exercise for seven to ten minutes, high-intensity, with thirty seconds of recovery, and that it does absolute wonders for your overall level of fitness, your oxygen utilization, weight loss, and strength. One HIIT in particular, the Scientific Seven-Minute Workout, includes a free mobile app, and is based on research done at the Human Performance Institute in Orlando, Florida. This mobile app is available through all app stores.

Whatever you decide to do, keep in mind that it only takes about three weeks to form a new habit. After years of self-neglect, in only twenty-one days you can begin to form a habit of exercise that can make a difference for the rest of your life.

## What's My Workout?

**This is what I do, mixing up the routine often:**

→ walking four to five times/week

→ walking with weights/rucking

→ Nordic Track ski machine

→ weight machines/free weights

→ mountain bike/trail riding

→ elliptical trainer

→ rowing machine

→ "Insanity"—warm-up and limited parts of the program

→ seven-minute workout

→ hiking any time I get a chance

→ medicine ball workout

# Make Exercise a Family Activity

Most of my patients have family. They have somebody else in their life: a significant other, a spouse, children, siblings, in-laws, a best friend. Whenever we talk to patients, we're also talking to the other people in the room because everyone is going to benefit from a change in lifestyle to include wellness. Getting on a low-salt diet, avoiding fast food, avoiding processed food, eating more vegetables and a plant-based diet is not just a program for the patient. We're not expecting patients to have to eat broccoli all day while someone else in the family is eating burgers and fries.

That includes exercise. We want exercise to become a family activity. Everyone in the family has to realize that going out and exercising, riding a bike together, going hiking, spending time together, is not only helping them, but it's helping the person that may need it more than them. That really is the key: Everyone must rally around the person that needs the help.

Good health and wellness takes planning. Meals must be planned, exercise must be planned. If you're just trying to fit everything in, that's not going to work. It all must be planned, and it must be planned with family and support.

# RAISE YOUR HEALTH IQ

1.  Using your hand, how large is a serving of meat?

2.  What is the best exercise to lose weight?

3.  What are the health benefits of hiking?

4.  How many steps per day are recommended for optimal health?

5.  What is sarcopenia?

# CHAPTER 10

# We Walk
# the Walk

→ *The Patient Experience*
→ *It's All about Patients*

**For more than** twenty-five years, I've taken care of people with liver disease, and in that time, I've seen fatty liver evolve to the point where it is now understood to be part of a bigger public health problem—namely, metabolic syndrome with all of its associated complications. While my team and I are experts on liver disease—including fatty liver, viral hepatitis (hepatitis B and hepatitis C), cirrhosis, liver cancer, and evaluating patients for liver transplant—by association, we are being forced to address the issues of obesity, eating disorders, and a lack of understanding of the foods people need to stay healthy.

At the recent American Association for the Study of Liver Diseases (AASLD) annual conference, there was an overwhelming amount of research and dialogue about fatty liver disease. Talks centered on new drug therapies that are in the FDA approval pipeline, new imaging technologies, and a greater understanding of the microbiome in the intestines that I discussed in chapter one.

Almost every presenter also talked about how to approach patients: How do we get patients to eat better food? To exercise? To commit to a lifestyle change? As physicians, they all understood the science, the biology, but they were mystified about who was going to attack the obesity epidemic and educate patients. I just listened because that's what I am doing with my practice. I am dedicating myself to addressing the issues that everyone else is talking about.

While the entire field of fatty liver disease has advanced where the science is concerned, it is still falling short when it comes to talking with patients and giving them guidance. It is still lacking in its ability to empower patients to be responsible for their health and make the changes to avoid a disastrous outcome with advancing liver disease, diabetes, heart disease, cancer, and other health problems. A life filled with multiple medical complications that could have been prevented by better personal decisions and food choices is simply unacceptable. We are *eating ourselves sick.*

That is the focal point of my practice, Liver Specialists of Texas and the Metabolic and Fatty Liver Center.

## The Patient Experience

In the previous chapters, I shared solutions that you can adopt for yourself and your family. But when the problems are more advanced, our team at the Metabolic and Fatty Liver Center can help.

Many patients who arrive at my practice already know that they have the diseases associated with metabolic syndrome. Sometimes they arrive after having put all the pieces together for themselves. They may have been told that they have high blood pressure, prediabetes, or high cholesterol. They know they're overweight and have truncal obesity. They may have even been diagnosed with fatty liver. But the information is organized in a disjointed fashion: Their primary care physician told them they're overweight. A cardiologist told them they have high blood pressure and cholesterol elevation and may have started treating them with a statin. An endocrinologist calmly told them they were prediabetic. As many as three different physicians may have mentioned the elements of metabolic syndrome, but no one tied it all together. No one told them about the risks they face and the long-term complications, and the likelihood of dying prematurely from this. No one gave them a cohesive plan for moving forward, because they assumed another provider would handle that. By the time these patients get to my door, they may have already begun to develop cirrhosis and more serious complications. It is this disjointed care patients receive that I find most distressing.

Whatever stage of the disease, the consultation at my practice begins by taking a detailed look at medical records. We want to go back several years to look at everything that's been done: scans, imaging, biopsies, surgical operative reports, and other therapies that the patient has undergone. We want to look at elements such as liver chemistries today versus two or five years ago. We want to know what imaging tests have found. For example, was fatty liver there five years ago? We want to know what other providers have found, and what plans have been offered. Even if that information is fragmented, our goal is to get a better understanding of our patients' health timeline and the sequence of events that brought them to the practice, and then to begin creating a coordinated effort.

We also take a detailed dietary history that includes our patients' social situation: What stressors or mitigating factors in their life are causing them to eat out? Do they travel for work? Are they a single parent? Are they on a limited budget? We want to know what they're eating, how they're eating, their favorite foods, and any food dislikes or allergies so we can start understanding what kind of plan to implement.

The evaluation includes studies related to the patients' body's characteristics. We measure height and weight, and then calculate body mass index. We measure body composition and get a sense of not only where the patients are today, but also how their body has changed. We look at the location of body fat—if it's centrally located—and then we want to see what can be done about reducing that belly fat or truncal obesity.

Members of our team determine a baseline assessment of balance, strength, conditioning, mobility, and flexibility. Part of the program includes recommendations on exercise and physical fitness, so we need to get a sense of what our patients are capable of doing.

The comprehensive physical examination also looks at heart, lung, and liver function, any sort of digestive issues, and any other factors that could potentially complicate our patients' progress.

From there, the evaluation moves to the laboratory, where comprehensive testing looks for other causes of liver problems such as genetic or hereditary forms of liver disease. We test for hepatitis C and want to know whether our patients have been vaccinated for hepatitis A and hepatitis B. The tests also look for other genetic disorders such as iron overload or hemochromatosis (discussed earlier in the book), along with screenings for diabetes, triglycerides, and cholesterol levels. Considering most individuals with metabolic syndrome die from the complications of cardiovascular disease, a detailed analysis and risk stratification of cardiovascular risks is also performed.

Other technologies used for testing may include ultrasound, a noninvasive test using sound waves that can diagnose fatty liver. It requires no preparation and can be done in the office. Ultrasound can also evaluate surrounding structures, including the gallbladder, pancreas, kidneys, and other abdominal organs. Whenever possible, we also use another non-invasive test called FibroScan (see chapter four) to calculate the degree of damage and/or fibrosis within the liver.

For some patients, there may also be associated emotional and psychological concerns to assess. Obesity is often the result of eating disorders, addiction, depression, anxiety, or problems with adjusting socially. Being evaluated by a mental health professional, as part of our team, is a useful facet of the evaluation process we have established.

In addition, for many patients, a physician-managed weight-loss program includes dietary planning, meal replacements, a customized exercise and fitness plan, and ongoing monitoring and follow-up, as needed. This program includes opportunities to participate in clinical trials, predominantly for new medicines that are being approved by the FDA for fatty liver disease.

For some patients, there is also an important discussion about bariatric surgery. That's why it's so crucial to get diagnosed early. Bariatric surgery may be an early intervention option. But with aggressive management of diet, exercise, weight loss, diabetes, and hyperlipidemia, bariatric surgery can often be averted.

Again, timing is everything in the realm of metabolic syndrome, fatty liver disease, and cirrhosis. There is a very definite cutoff point where it's no longer safe to perform any form of bariatric or weight reduction surgery on a patient with liver cirrhosis. However, these days, some centers are actually performing liver transplant and bariatric surgery at the same time in an effort to help patients keep from regaining weight post-transplant. Twenty years ago, that would never have been considered, but with the rising rate of obesity, we are all being forced to be more aggressive with our patients.

## It's All about Patients

Once I knew I was going to be a physician, even before I entered medical school, I had a dream of how my practice would operate: I wanted to have exceptional physician/patient relationships. That may be the most meaningful part of my job and why I get up every morning, and head to work.

Every day, I want patients to truly realize that I am there for them. Period. It's all about trying to make them healthier and reduce their disease. While I do this partly because of my own experiences with family or friends, the desire to help all patients comes from deep in my heart.

Since there's only one of me, and so many patients to see, I have to rely on very well trained staff to help me fulfill my dream. At Liver Specialists of Texas and the Metabolic and Fatty Liver Center, we invest in training our staff in the latest technology, research, and therapies. We also spend time talking about why they do what they do, and why communication is so vital to their role. I pride myself on being a physician communicator, so I challenge my staff to also be the best communicators they can be.

At all times, we also stress the importance of great customer service. As I mentioned earlier in this book, getting service from a doctor these days is the same as anywhere else you shop or have person-to-person interactions. You want the person you're working with to deliver a high level of value.

We also work tirelessly on patient education in a very caring fashion. I believe that's critical to making our patients well. When patients understand what is wrong and why their situation is bad, they better understand the level of danger they are in and are more motivated to take responsibility for their own health. We believe knowledge is power, and early intervention means fewer complications.

Why did I title this chapter "We Walk the Walk"? Because that's what I do. When I tell patients to eat better, and exercise, cook at home more, be organized and a smart shopper, entertain at home, it's because I do those things myself. So, I don't feel the least bit guilty in telling you to do it too!

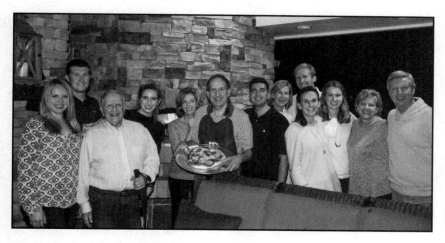

Dr. Galati cooking for his family and friends.

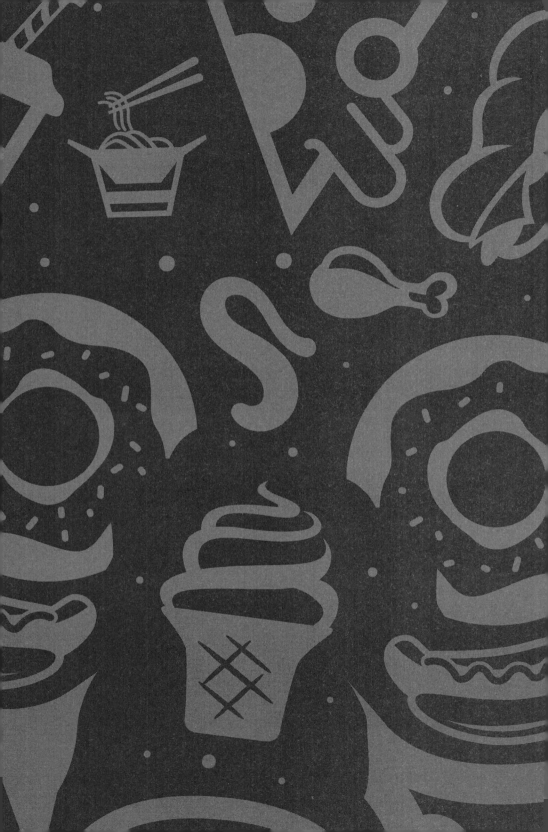

# CONCLUSION

# No Excuses—
# "You Gotta'
# Wanna' Do It"

**Recently, I participated** in an art exhibit in Houston, in which I displayed a large collection of my photography. I've been a photographer most of my life, and have amassed a fairly large collection. I was one of twenty-eight physicians who are also artists; it was an opportunity for the people of Houston to see a group of physicians who were not only leaders in their field, but were also human being, without white coats.

A large crowd of Houstonians showed up for the one-night event, one of which was an older gentleman who spent a few minutes talking with me. He was an engineer who owned his own company, and he told me he couldn't believe I had a collection of photos on display that spanned a nearly forty-year time frame. In the sincerest way, he marveled at the fact that I was able to participate in the show and have so many pieces on display considering how busy I am as a physician, how much time I've spent getting a medical education, and the fact that, on the side, I have also been doing a radio show for fifteen years. "You are an inspiration for anybody that says they don't have the time to do something," he told me.

That's the message I hope you take away from this book.

People regularly tell me they don't have time to exercise, they don't have time to cook, they don't have time to clean up after preparing a meal, they don't have time to take interest in their own health. But I'm onto you—those are all very weak excuses.

If you want to excel in anything, you can do it—there's absolutely no reason you can't. But as my father always taught me, first, "You gotta' wanna' do it."

When it comes to your physical well-being, it takes time and commitment, but it is not impossible. However, if you spend all your time making excuses instead, then you're going to have a very tough time—and there's really nobody to blame but yourself. Everyone says: "I don't have time." I say, "Make time."

Now is the time to take metabolic syndrome, obesity, fatty liver disease, diabetes, and heart disease seriously. Society is at the point, both in the United States and globally, where obesity is affecting not only adults, but also children. As a parent, letting yourself go is one thing, but think about your kids and their futures. The habits you're instilling in them today are going to handicap them as adults. As parents, grandparents, educators, coaches—we are responsible for kids today. This is just too important to not take seriously. It's time to say enough is enough.

If you're a parent, you're going to have to take a stand. You've got to fight popular culture and peer pressure. You've got to become the unpopular mom or dad who doesn't have junk food in the house or who eats Happy Meals after sports. You've got to forego some of the more meaningless things in life to make time to plan, shop healthy, and cook. This is about your family, and it's about your future. As I discussed in the opening paragraphs of the book, my mother was the first up every morning making sure we all had a fresh, healthy breakfast to start the day. Her never ending drive to make sure we ate well—for the sake of her family's health—was admirable fifty years ago, and I believe we need to make it the standard operating procedure again today.

Everything trickles down from wellness. If we don't get a handle on it in this country, the economic impact is going to be debilitating.

But if we have a well society, with fit young children—with people who are well nourished, free of chronic progressive diseases—then everyone and everything will perform better. That means fewer doctor visits, fewer missed work or school days, and people who are more creative doers and shakers. In short, we're going to be a more successful country as a whole.

I put this book together in hopes of enlightening you. I want you to realize it's not too late to change, it's not too late to get back on track. And it doesn't really take much effort if you want to make the change.

Metabolic syndrome is a very winnable battle, not only for yourself but the rest of your family. There are just a handful of new skills and habits you need to gradually implement over time to get you back on track to health, vitality, and the prevention of disease. I've seen it for myself in many patients for whom one or two adjustments made all the difference in the world. You can do it, too. You must make the commitment to succeed.

# Our Services

Liver Specialists of Texas and the Metabolic and Fatty Liver Center provides a wide range of specialized care to patients with digestive and liver disorders. Dr. Joseph S. Galati has been practicing in the Texas Medical Center since 1994.

Center staff includes:

➜     Hepatologists  (liver specialists)

➜     Gastroenterologists

➜     Nutritionists and dieticians

➜     Exercise physiologist and trainers

➜     Psychologist

➜     Psychiatrist

➜     Bariatric surgeon

➜     Endocrinologist

Our warm, receptive staff is available for all your needs. A comprehensive evaluation at the center begins with detailed medical histories and includes a thorough physical examination, lab testing, and more.

Patients requiring hospitalization for more complicated problems are treated in the adjacent Houston Methodist Hospital, one of the nation's leading hospitals and one of the finest hospitals in the Texas Medical Center.

Same-day procedures, such as liver biopsies, upper endoscopies, and colonoscopies, are performed on an outpatient basis at the Texas International Endoscopy Center.

The comprehensive care provided by Dr. Galati and team address include the following disorders and services:

## Disorders

➔ Non-alcoholic fatty liver disease
➔ Viral hepatitis
➔ Alcoholic liver disease
➔ Hepatitis C
➔ Hepatitis B
➔ Cirrhosis
➔ Portal hypertension
➔ Gastrointestinal bleeding
➔ Liver cancer
➔ Hemochromatosis/iron overload
➔ Autoimmune hepatitis
➔ Liver failure
➔ Liver transplantation

## Services

➔ Weight loss management
➔ Nutritional assessment and support
➔ Exercise/physical assessment
➔ Liver biopsy
➔ Colonoscopy and colon cancer screening
➔ Upper endoscopy
➔ Banding of esophageal varices
➔ Liver transplantation
➔ Paracentesis
➔ Liver ultrasound
➔ FibroScan
➔ Clinical research participation

**For more information, go to www.drjoegalati.com.**

# ABOUT THE AUTHOR

**Dr. Joseph S. Galati,** a native of Long Island, New York, was raised in a family where good nutrition and family were ways of life. Today, his practice, Liver Specialists of Texas and the Metabolic and Fatty Liver Center, is devoted to the care of patients with all facets of liver diseases, obesity, fatty liver, and nutrition-related disorders.

After medical school at St. George's University of Medicine, he pursued further training in Internal Medicine at SUNY-Health Science Center-Brooklyn/Kings County Hospital Center and further expertise in Liver Disease and Transplant Medicine at the University of Nebraska Medical Center, one of the finest liver centers in the country.

Dr. Galati has been involved in clinical research in liver disease for the past thirty years, conducting studies in viral hepatitis and non-alcoholic fatty liver disease. A Fellow in the American Association for the Study of Liver Diseases and American College of Gastroenterology, Dr. Galati has been an invited speaker both nationally and internationally, having lectured in Latin America, Europe, and Asia. He is a Diplomat in the American Board of Internal Medicine-Gastroenterology. Currently, Dr. Galati is the Medical Director of the Sherrie and Alan Conover Center for Liver Disease & Transplantation at Houston Methodist Hospital, one of the finest hospitals and research institutes in the United States.

He is the founder of Your Health First Education, a 501(c)(3) organization whose mission is to provide education and support to the public, raising awareness about liver disease, obesity, alcohol abuse, nutrition, disease screening, and early intervention.

Since 2003, Dr. Galati has created consumer-oriented radio programming on health and wellness, producing and hosting "Your Health First," a one-hour radio program each weekend, heard on iHeart Radio's 740 am KTRH, and streamed globally on the iHeart app.

When not practicing medicine, Dr. Galati is an avid photographer, outdoors enthusiast, and is a board member of Entrepreneur's Organization, supporting entrepreneurs in all corners of the world. Dr. Galati and his wife, Geraldine, are active with several Houston charities, and have two children, Joseph and Elizabeth.

**For more information about Dr. Joe Galati, please visit www.drjoegalati.com**

# ENDNOTES

1   "The IDF Consensus Worldwide Definition of the Metabolic Syndrome," International Diabetes Federation, 2006.

2   "Obesity and Overweight," World Health Organization, June 2016, accessed September 2017, http://www.who.int/mediacentre/factsheets/fs311/en.

3   Ibid.

4   "Obesity Rates and Trends Overview," The State of Obesity, accessed September 2017, https://stateofobesity.org/obesity-rates-trends-overview.

5   Ibid.

6   "Obesity and overweight," World Health Organization, June 2016, accessed September 2017, http://www.who.int/mediacentre/factsheets/fs311/en.

7   Zachary J. Ward, "Simulation of Growth Trajectories of Childhood Obesity into Adulthood," *The New England Journal of Medicine* 377 (November 2017): 2145–2153, https://doi.org/10.1056/NEJMoa1703860

8   "10 Reasons America Is Morbidly Obese," Salon.com, August 1, 2014, accessed September 2017, http://www.salon.com/2014/08/01/10_reasons_america_is_morbidly_obese_partner.

9   Ibid.

10  Ibid.

11  Ibid.

12  Franklin Tsai and Walter J. Coyle, "The Microbiome and Obesity: Is Obesity Linked to Our Gut Flora?" *Current Gastroenterology Reports* 11 (2009): 307–313.

13  Clarisse A. Marotz and Amir Zarrinpar, "Treating Obesity and Metabolic Syndrome with Fecal Microbiota Transplantation," Yale J Biol Med 89, no. 3 (September 2016): 383–388, https://www.ncbi.nlm.nih.gov/pmc/articles/PMC5045147/

14 Michaeleen Doucleff, "Is the Secret to a Healthier Microbiome Hidden in the Hadza Diet?" NPR, August 24, 2017, accessed September 2017, http://www.npr.org/sections/goatsandso-da/2017/08/24/545631521/is-the-secret-to-a-healthier-micro-biome-hidden-in-the-hadza-diet?utm_medium=RSS&utm_campaign=world.

15 "The IDF Consensus Worldwide Definition of the Metabolic Syn-drome," International Diabetes Federation, 2006.

16 "Statistics about Diabetes," American Diabetes Association, accessed September 2017, http://www.diabetes.org/diabetes-basics/statistics.

17 Ibid.

18 "The IDF Consensus Worldwide Definition of the Metabolic Syn-drome," International Diabetes Federation, 2006.

19 "Weight Problems Take a Hefty Toll on Body and Mind," Harvard T. H. Chan School of Public Health, Obesity Prevention Source, accessed September 14, 2017, https://www.hsph.harvard.edu/obesity-prevention-source/obesity-consequences/health-effects.

20 Hashem El-Serag, "The Association between Obesity and GERD: A Review of the Epidemiological Evidence," *Digestive Diseases and Sciences* 53, no. 9 (September 2008): 2307–2312, accessed September 11, 2017, https://doi.org/10.1007/s10620-008-0413-9

21 Ibid.

22 Abel Romero-Corral et al., "Interactions between Obesity and Ob-structive Sleep Apnea," *CHEST* 137, no. 3 (March 2010): 711–719, https://doi.org/10.1378/chest.09-0360

23 Ibid.

24 Ibid.

25 Emily Jungheim et al., "Obesity and Reproductive Function," *Ob-stetrics and Gynecology Clinics of North America* 39, no. 4 (December 2012): 479–493, https://doi.org/10.1016/j.ogc.2012.09.002

26 John Brannian, "Obesity and Fertility," *South Dakota Medicine* 64, no. 7 (July 2011): 251–254, https://www.ncbi.nlm.nih.gov/pubmed/21848022

27   "Weight Problems Take a Hefty Toll on Body and Mind," Harvard T. H. Chan School of Public Health, accessed September 2017, https:// www.hsph.harvard.edu/obesity-prevention-source/obesity-conse-quences/health-effects; Ivana Vucenik and Joseph Stains, "Obesity and Cancer Risk: Evidence, Mechanisms, and Recommendations," *Annuls of the New York Academy of Sciences* 1271, (2012): 37–43, https://doi.org/10.1111/j.1749-6632.2012.06750.x

28   Neil Iyengar et al., "Obesity and Cancer Mechanisms: Tumor Microenvironment and Inflammation," *Journal of Clinical Oncology* 34, no. 35 (December 2016): 4210–4276, https://doi.org/10.1200/ JCO.2016.67.4283

29   Genevieve Gariepy et al., "The Interaction of Obesity and Psycholog-ical Distress on Disability," *Social Psychiatry and Psychiatric Epidemiol-ogy* 45, no. 5 (2010): 531–540, https://doi.org/10.1007/s00127-009-0090-9

30   Munim Mannan et al., "Prospective Associations between Depres-sion and Obesity for Adolescent Males and Females: A Systematic Review and Meta-Analysis of Longitudinal Studies," *PLOS One* (June 10, 2016): 1–18.

31   Kenneth Thorpe, "The Future Costs of Obesity: National and State Estimates of the Impact of Obesity on Direct Healthcare Expenses," National Collaborative on Childhood Obesity Research, November 2009, accessed September 2017, http://nccor.org/downloads/Costo-fObesityReport-FINAL.pdf.

32   Ibid.

33   Maximillian Tremmel et al., "Economic Burden of Obesity: A Systematic Literature Review," *International Journal of Environmental Research and Public Health* 14, no. 435 (2017): 1–18.

34   Eric Finkelstein et al., "The Costs of Obesity among Full-Time Em-ployees," *American Journal of Health Promotion* 20, no. 1 (September/ October 2005): 45–51.

35   Ibid.

36   Rolan Sturm, Jeanne Ringel, and Tatiana Andreyeva, "Increas-ing Obesity Rates and Disability Trends," *Health Affairs* 21, no. 2 (March/April 2004): 199–203.

37   C. M. Teuner et al., "Impact of BMI and BMI Change on Future Drug Expenditures in Adults: Results from the MON-ICA/KORA Cohort Study," *BMC Health Services Research* 13 (424), 2013.

38   Ibid.

39   Kenneth Thorpe, "The Future Costs of Obesity: National and State Estimates of the Impact of Obesity on Direct Healthcare Expenses," National Collaborative on Childhood Obesity Research, November 2009, accessed September 2017, http://nccor.org/downloads/CostofObesityReport-FINAL.pdf.

40   Beth Baker, "The Enormous Economic Costs of America's Obesity Epidemic," *The Week,* April 9, 2017. "Statistics about Diabetes," American Diabetes Association, accessed September 2017, http://www.diabetes.org/diabetes-basics/statistics.

41   Arpita Tiwari et al., "Cooking at Home: A Strategy to Comply With U.S. Dietary Guidelines at No Extra Cost," *American Journal of Preventative Medicine* 52, no. 5 (May 2017): 616–624, https://doi.org/10.1016/
j.amepre.2017.01.017

42   Maria Lamagna, "Why millennials don't know how to cook," Personal Finance, MarketWatch, last modified September 10, 2016, https://www.marketwatch.com/story/why-millennials-dont-know-how-to-cook-2016-08-10

43   "11 Facts About American Eating Habits," DoSomething.org, https://www.dosomething.org/us/facts/11-facts-about-american-eating-habits

44   Bruce Weitz, answer on the question, "What Product Categories Generate Most Volume In A Grocery Store?" Quora, August 7, 2013, https://www.forbes.com/sites/quora/2013/08/07/what-product-cate-gories-generate-most-volume-in-a-grocery-store/#682e0683d32b

45   Neil Howe, "Millennials Struggle to Pass Life Skills 101," Forbes, last modified July 2, 2014, https://www.forbes.com/sites/neilhowe/2014/07/02/millennials-struggle-to-pass-life-skills-101/#1d23651f79e7

46   Clinical Practice Guidelines, "EASL–EASD–EASO Clinical Practice Guidelines for the Management

of Non-Alcoholic Fatty Liver Disease." *EASL Journal of Hepatology* 66, no. 2: 465–466, accessed September 12, 2017, http://www.easl.eu/medias/cpg/2016-04/EASL_CPG-NAFLD.pdf.

47   C. Lam, F. E. Murray, and A. Cuschieri, *"Increased Cholecystectomy Rate after the Introduction of Laparoscopic Cholecystectomy in Scotland,"* *Gut* 38 (1996): 282–284.

48   Petros Zezos and Eberhard Renner, "Liver Transplantation and Non-Alcoholic Fatty Liver Disease," *World Journal of Gastroenterology* 20, no. 42 (November 14, 2014): 15532–15538.

49   Ibid.

50   "Liver Competing Risk Percentage with Deceased Donor Transplant at Specific Time Points for Registrations Listed: 2003–2014, based on OPTN data as of November 24, 2017," Organ Procurement and Transplantation Network, US Department of Health and Human Services, accessed November 29, 2017, https://optn.transplant.hrsa.gov/data/view-data-reports/national-data.

51   Gloria Sin, "Microsoft: Almost 25 Percent of Computers Are Still Unprotected from Viruses and Malware," *Digital Trends*, April 18, 2013.

52   "CDC: Adult Vaccination Rates Are Drastically Low," Fox News, February 7, 2014, accessed October 2, 2017, http://www.foxnews.com/health/2014/02/07/cdc-adult-vaccination-rates-are-drastically-low.html.

53   The Global BMI Mortality Collaboration, "Body-Mass Index and All-Cause Mortality: Individual Participant-Data Meta-Analysis of 239 Prospective Studies in Four Continents," *The Lancet* 388 (August 20, 2016): 776–786.

54   "Cholesterol Levels: What You Need to Know," NIH MedlinePlus, accessed October 7, 2017, https://medlineplus.gov/magazine/issues/summer12/articles/summer12pg6-7.html.

55   CDC, "More than 100 Million Americans Have Diabetes or Pre-diabetes," press release, July 18, 2017, https://www.cdc.gov/media/releases/2017/p0718-diabetes-report.html

56  Paul Kwo, Stanley M. Cohen, and Joseph K. Lim, "ACG Practice Guideline: Evaluation of Abnormal Liver Chemistries," *The American Journal of Gastroenterology* 112, no. 1 (2016): 18–35.

57  Rebecca Rupp, "Surviving the Sneaky Psychology of Supermarkets," *National Geographic*, June 15, 2015, accessed October 5, 2017, http://theplate.nationalgeographic.com/2015/06/15/surviving-the-sneaky-psychology-of-supermarkets.

58  "Guidance for Industry: A Food Labeling Guide (8. Claims)," US Food and Drug Administration, January 2013, accessed October 8, 2017, https://www.fda.gov/Food/GuidanceRegulation/GuidanceDocumentsRegulatoryInformation/LabelingNutrition/ucm064908.htm.

59  "Ibid.

60  "Correct Portion Sizes: How to Keep Portion Distortion in Check," Dairy Council of California, accessed October 6, 2017, https://www.healthyeating.org/Healthy-Eating/Healthy-Living/Weight-Management/Article-Viewer/Article/348/correct-portion-sizes-how-to-keep-portion-distortion-in-check.

61  "Serving-Size Chart," Dairy Council of California, accessed October 6, 2017, https://www.healthyeating.org/Portals/0/Documents/Schools/Parent%20Ed/Portion_Sizes_Serving_Chart.pdf?ver=2017-08-31-150411-207.

62  "Food Serving Sizes Get a Reality Check," US Food and Drug Administration, accessed October 6, 2017, https://www.fda.gov/For-Consumers/ConsumerUpdates/ucm386203.htm.

63  Information on storing vegetables and fruit can be found on the Fruits and Veggies More Matters website at https://www.fruitsandveggiesmorematters.org/wp-content/uploads/UserFiles/File/pdf/why/Storing_Fruits_Veggies_FINAL.pdf.

64  Aamer Madhani, "Treadmill Injuries Send Thousands to the ER Every Year," *USA Today*, May 5, 2014.

65  Gale Bernhardt, "The Real Reason You Should Warm Up," Active.com, accessed September 2017, https://www.active.com/triathlon/articles/the-real-reason-you-should-warm-up

66   Markham Heid, "Why Hiking Is the Perfect Mind-Body Workout," *Time*, July 5, 2017.

67   Ibid.

68   "How Much Physical Activity Do Adults Need?" Centers for Disease Control and Prevention, accessed November 11, 2017, https://www.cdc.gov/physicalactivity/basics/adults/index.htm.

69   "Sarcopenia with Aging," WebMD, accessed November 11, 2017, https://www.webmd.com/healthy-aging/guide/sarcopenia-with-aging#1.

70   Courtenay Dunn-Lewis and William Kraemer, "The Basics of Starting and Progressing a Strength-Training Program," American College of Sports Medicine, October 7, 2016, accessed January 18, 2017, http://www.acsm.org/public-information/articles/2016/10/07/the-basics-of-starting-and-progressing-a-strength-training-program.

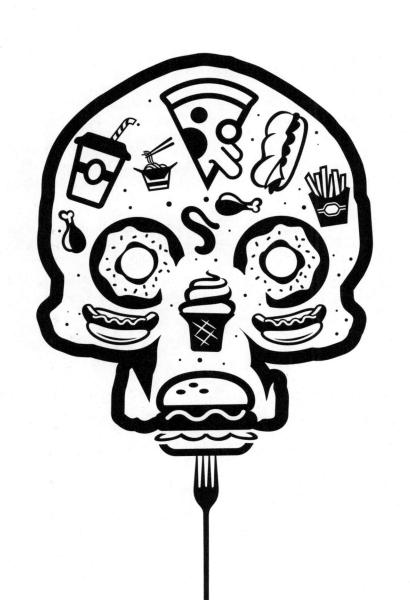

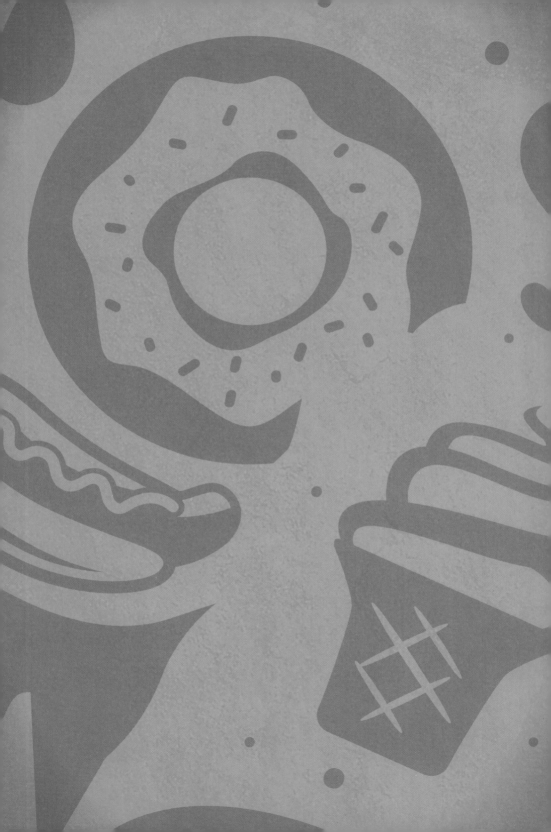